T0227905

CULTURAL FACTORS IN DELINQUENCY

TAVISTOCK

CRIME & DELINQUENCY
In 10 Volumes

CULTURAL FACTORS IN DELINQUENCY

EDITED BY T C N GIBBENS AND
R H AHRENFELDT

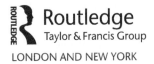

Routledge
Taylor & Francis Group

LONDON AND NEW YORK

First published in 1966 by
Tavistock Publications Limited

Published in 2001 by
Routledge
2 Park Square, Milton Park, Abingdon, Oxfordshire OX14 4RN
711 Third Avenue, New York, NY 10017

First issued in paperback 2014

Routledge is an imprint of the Taylor and Francis Group, an informa business

British Library Cataloguing in Publication Data
A CIP catalogue record for this book
is available from the British Library

Cultural Factors in Delinquency
ISBN 0-415-26411-1
Crime & Delinquency: 10 Volumes
ISBN 0-415-26507-X
The International Behavioural and Social Sciences Library
112 Volumes
ISBN 0-415-25670-4

ISBN 13: 978-1-138-86135-0 (pbk)
ISBN 13: 978-0-415-26411-2 (hbk)

Cultural Factors in Delinquency

Edited by

T. C. N. GIBBENS, M.A., M.D., D.P.M.
Reader in Forensic Psychiatry, University of London

and

R. H. AHRENFELDT, M.R.C.S., L.R.C.P.
Consultant and Research Associate, World Federation for Mental Health

TAVISTOCK PUBLICATIONS

J. B. LIPPINCOTT COMPANY

First published in 1966
by Tavistock Publications Limited
2 Park Square, Milton Park, Abingdon, Oxon, OX14 4RN
This book has been set in 10 on 12 pt Modern Extended
The Camelot Press Ltd, Southampton
© *World Federation for Mental Health, 1966*

Distributed in Canada and the United States
of America
by J. B. Lippincott Company
Philadelphia and Montreal

CONTENTS

PREFACE

by

Dr John R. Rees

Hon. President, World Federation for Mental Health

Since its foundation in 1948, the World Federation has constantly had in mind the problems arising from delinquency as something demanding study. It was felt, however, that the topic had been covered pretty well by the International Society and, of course, by the Social Defence Section of the United Nations.

Shortly before I ceased to be the Director of the Federation, the suggestion came, primarily from Dr Otto Klineberg, that we might well look into the question of the cultural factors and their contribution to the whole problem of delinquency. Since it had been raised at that point, my successor in the Federation asked me if I would carry on the original plan of bringing the group together, which I did with much pleasure; and we assembled an international group from sixteen countries and a considerable number of separate disciplines to discuss the theme of this report. It may have been a little disappointing to some that we did not find more new material about the effects of peer groups and their opportunities of learning and unlearning delinquent behaviour, but it was clear that there were so many unknown factors and problems which needed to be tackled in the statistical field all over the world before we could get much further, that this coloured the thinking of the study group.

The study group meeting was held at Topeka, Kansas by the generous invitation of the Menninger Foundation. In organizing this group, we had the very great help of the Aquinas Fund of America in providing support for the preliminary work by Dr R. H. Ahrenfeldt in surveying the existing literature; and the major costs of the group meeting, its travel costs, etc., were met by the Maurice Falk Medical Fund of Pittsburgh, through the efforts of the United States Committee of the Federation. To these, who did so much to make the effort possible, we owe a great debt of gratitude; and at the moment it is appropriate to say how enormously indebted we are to Dr Robert Ahrenfeldt and Dr Trevor Gibbens for their

ix

thoughtful help and consistent work. Dr Gibbens, as a leading criminologist, acted as our consultant, but he was much more than this, for he became rapporteur, as well as being now the main editor of this report. The good things that were found to come out of the study group's work are largely the result of the thought and work of these two physicians.

EDITORS' INTRODUCTION

In making this report of the transactions of the Topeka Conference on Cultural Factors in Delinquency, the editors have been obliged to depart from the usual practice. Many reports of this kind publish the basic document or documents supplied to the participants, and go on to provide a verbatim, if edited, version of the discussion. This often results in a rather diffuse treatment of the subject, with particular topics being mentioned in several widely separated places in the text. This method undoubtedly extracts the maximum information from a conference, but it has the disadvantage of being very time-consuming. It requires one or two years to edit transactions of this kind and submit to each participant, for his approval, a version of what he has contributed. For several reasons it was thought better to prepare the present report within a limited time and, in consequence, the editors have had to take a heavy responsibility for its contents.

The participants discussed the subject in the same order as the present chapter headings, with the help of a preliminary document prepared by Dr Ahrenfeldt. The contents of this document with many additions suggested by the conference have been dispersed throughout the report, incorporating the comments and arguments of the participants. Since these comments are not given verbatim and in order to avoid misrepresentation, those who made them are not mentioned by name unless we were able to refer to available publications that developed the same arguments or points of view. Those who wish to follow up their line of thought are referred to the bibliography. The reader should bear in mind, therefore, that any particular observation or opinion may have been either included in the original document, or contributed during the conference (not necessarily by the representative of the relevant country), or else subsequently extracted from the literature.

Editing and selecting the points raised in discussion have placed a heavy burden upon the editors, and we apologize in advance to any participants who feel that their comments have been ignored or not given sufficient emphasis. Since the meeting was composed of sociologists, lawyers, criminologists, psychiatrists, psychologists, and anthropologists, it is inevitable that there should be some different views, but all the participants will probably agree that the extent to which the different disciplines were able to communicate with one another in a most harmonious way under the skilled chairmanship of Professor Otto Klineberg was one of the outstanding features of the conference. If this report conveys some impression of the degree of mutual understanding, and the active collaboration achieved by the representatives of different disciplines and different countries, the editors will feel fully rewarded.

It hardly needs to be stressed that the cultural aspects of delinquency cover a vast area of study. It would have been quite impossible in the course of one week's discussion to make a comprehensive survey of this field. Our hope is that this review, short as it is, will provide the reader who has neither the time nor the specialized knowledge to study the vast literature with a deeper insight into the complex and important problems involved.

T. C. N. GIBBENS
R. H. AHRENFELDT

ACKNOWLEDGEMENTS

The Editors and all who took part in the Topeka Conference wish to express their deep gratitude to the Falk Medical Fund of Pittsburgh, and its President, Mr Philip Hallen, for financial support for the meeting; to the Aquinas Fund of America for support for the preparation of the preliminary document; to the World Federation for Mental Health through its Honorary President, Dr J. R. Rees; to Professor Otto Klineberg, late Chairman of the Federation's Executive Board and its next President, both for his initiation of the concept and for his splendid chairmanship of the group; and also to Mr William T. Beaty, the Director of the Federation's New York office, whose tireless efforts succeeded in gathering us together; and to the Menninger Foundation for its hospitality.

Thanks are due to the individuals and publishers concerned for permission to quote passages from the following works:
The American Academy of Political and Social Science in respect of 'Resocialization within Walls' by L. W. McCorkle and R. Korn from *The Annals*, 1954; the author and the editors of *The British Journal of Criminology* in respect of 'The Soviet Law of Commissions for Cases of Juveniles' by R. Beermann; Messrs T. & T. Clark in respect of Hastings' *Encyclopaedia of Religion and Ethics*, Vol. 12; Collins Publishers in respect of *The Honoured Society* by N. Lewis; E. P. Dutton & Co. in respect of *Shakespeare of London* by Marchette Chute; the Macmillan Company in respect of *Culture and Mental Disorders* by J. W. Eaton and R. J. Weil; Methuen & Co. Ltd in respect of *The Greek View of Life* by G. Lowes Dickinson; Routledge & Kegan Paul Ltd in respect of *Sex and Temperament in Three Primitive Societies* by Margaret Mead, and *Ethical Relativity* by E. Westermarck; the Trustees of the Institute for Sex Research and W. B. Saunders Company in respect of *Sexual Behavior in the Human Male* by A. C. Kinsey *et al.*; Social Science Research Council, New York, in respect of *Culture, Conflict, and Crime* by Thorsten Sellin; the authors and the editor of *Teachers College Record* in respect of 'Organization and Social Function of Japanese Gangs' by G. A. De Vos and K. Mizushima; the World Federation for Mental Health in respect of *Mental Health in International Perspective*.

PART ONE

Chapter 1

DEFINITIONS

Anyone who wishes to discuss the cultural factors in delinquency must first decide upon the scope and subject-matter of discussion. What are delinquency and crime? In many ways, the attempt to answer this question at once takes us to the heart of the problem. As Lord Atkin said in 1939, 'The domain of criminal jurisprudence can only be ascertained by examining what acts at any particular period are declared by the State to be crimes, and the only common nature they will be found to possess is that they are prohibited by the State and that those who commit them are punished' (Hall Williams, 1964). There are profound cultural differences between States and regional jurisdictions within States in the extent to which definitions arise from emotion or the views of a ruling class, in the speed of evolution from one 'particular period' to another, in the attitudes adopted to 'punishment'. These cultural differences, and the various factors influencing them, are the subject-matter of this report. We must begin by discussing the variety of definitions of crime.

There is nowadays substantial agreement between criminologists that they should not 'stray too far from the consideration of behaviour legally defined as criminal' (Hall Williams, 1964). Their essential subject-matter is the varieties of behaviour that are defined as delinquent by the criminal law. This does not mean, however, that criminologists must confine their attention to this aspect: it would in fact be prejudicial to any real advance if they were to do so. They have to develop a specific science of behaviour, and to make use of all that is already available in the behavioural sciences adequate to explain and interpret the acts that result in breaking the law. Unless we extend consideration to the types of *behaviour* which are illegal, and consider the motives for them and their social context, we cannot make any 'horizontal' comparison between one country or legal jurisdiction and another at the same point in time, nor can we make 'vertical' comparisons between one generation and another in a particular country. If attempted suicide, for example, ceases to be defined as a crime in a particular country, it does not thereby lose all interest for the social scientist or even the criminologist: he may still be concerned to study the trends in this form of behaviour.

The Topeka Conference was mainly concerned with juvenile delinquency; and there is little doubt that the problems of definition are much more complex in relation to juveniles than to adults. The newer and vaguer terms defining the type of behaviour which could bring a child before a juvenile court or similar tribunal – 'incorrigibility', being a 'wayward minor', 'in need of care or protection', 'in moral danger', 'beyond control', and so on – were probably introduced in order to remove juvenile delinquency from the scope of the adult criminal law and ensure that it was treated in a quite different way.

During the decade following the Second World War there was a strong movement in some international circles, e.g. at the First United Nations' Congress in Geneva in 1955 (United Nations, 1956), to belittle any attempt at a strict definition of delinquency. We are concerned, it was said, with 'disturbed' or 'maladjusted' children, with deprived, neglected 'pre-delinquents' who show a variety of behaviour disorders. Social and legal measures should be concentrated upon this essential problem; and whether some particular act would be defined in an adult as criminal was quite incidental and unimportant. More recently, however, the trend has been reversed. It is realized that, without prejudice to this wider understanding of children's needs, it is necessary *for certain purposes* to define delinquency as comprising certain kinds of behaviour disorder. The National Council on Crime and Delinquency, the Second United Nations' Congress (United Nations, 1960), and other bodies have recommended that delinquency should refer to acts which, if committed by an adult, would be regarded as criminal. This does not solve the problem but it comes closer to providing a criterion for use in the development of comparative studies.

Before dealing with the complexities of definition in juveniles, however, it is useful to point out the great variations that exist even in the definition of adult crime. These cultural variations exist equally in the case of juveniles, but with the added complication that the offender is subject to special attitudes and treatments because of his immature age (cf. Soddy, 1961).

4

The Definition of Adult Crime

The age at which a person is regarded as an adult by the criminal law varies, but from a cultural standpoint we may think of an adult as a mature person whom the vast majority of mature citizens would regard as 'one of themselves', responsible, as they are, for their illegal acts. This sense of identification with the offender, though often illusory to a greater or lesser extent, profoundly affects the way in which he is treated.

Crime is defined when a society with recognized norms of behaviour, or a part of society which has power and authority to do so, categorizes certain types of extreme or damaging behaviour as liable to punishment. The concept of crime seems inseparably linked to punishment, and usually, but not invariably, punishment by society rather than by the individual (early Scandinavian and English laws appear to have sometimes given a public licence, so to speak, for the victim to carry out private revenge of a socially approved type). Not all deviant behaviour is defined as crime; other deviations may perhaps be regarded as more in the nature of sins, unless they are mild enough to be tolerated eccentricities.

What happens, one may ask, in cultures which have never developed a criminal law? There must be contravention of mores. It may be that such cultures are particularly stable and homogeneous, and that the offender exiles himself. It is said that, in some Pacific islands, the murderer is left to go and hang himself, rather as the member of a rigid military caste who had dishonoured it was expected to shoot himself. Durkheim (1895), however, emphasized many years ago that there could be no society without crime; if it were reduced to a minimum then the largest deviations, however small, would come to be regarded as crimes. Biological variation would ensure this amount of deviation. In the devout atmosphere of a monastery, slackness, loss of zeal, or bad temper become subject to punishment as serious infractions. In fact, in mediaeval monasteries, the disease of *accidie*, a state of depressed boredom and loss of zeal resulting in the gabbling of prayers, etc., was considered a mortal sin (Power, 1922) and Dante allotted to them a special place in his *Inferno*. Durkheim maintained that the constructive aspects of progress and originality could not exist in a society without the misdirected initiative which constitutes crime. In our own

5

generation, in which a remarkably high proportion of the rulers of the world have spent some part of their lives in prison, his views have special force.

One of the most remarkable instances of a criminal code, evolved by a highly cohesive society in which virtually all the members are devoted to similar principles, is provided by the Penal Code established in Pennsylvania in 1682 by the Quakers under the leadership of William Penn (Barnes, 1927). The Duke of York's laws, promulgated for the American Colonies in 1664, provided the death penalty for those found guilty of blasphemy, murder, treason, homosexuality, bestiality, some forms of conspiracy, and for 'any child over 16 who strikes his natural father or mother except in defence of his life'. The law adopted by William Penn's first assembly in 1682, however, was 300 years ahead of its time; it is no accident that the Quakers have remained in the vanguard of penal reform. They abolished the death penalty for every crime but murder, abolished the grosser forms of corporal punishment, and substituted imprisonment as the punishment for the majority of serious offences. Breaking and entering and theft of goods, for example, were punishable by fourfold restitution and three months' imprisonment; or, if there were no restitution, by seven years' imprisonment. But, as in most homogeneous and highly cohesive societies, crime was regarded as very close to sin. Profanity, gambling, drunkenness, and even smoking in the streets were relatively severely punished. Sexual laxity, especially, was strongly repressed: even a married woman who had a baby less than nine months after marriage was liable to have her head shaved and to be made to stand in the pillory.

In the world today, there are a number of reasons for variations in the definition of criminal behaviour. The criminal law, since it must have the support of the majority of society, is always a conservative force. There are usually elements of the law which are obsolete; remaining in force, but no longer having an application to modern conditions. Also, the law is usually out of date in some respects in the sense that offences may be quite evident to society before they become legally defined as such. In a changing society such developments result in a considerable distinction being made between the concepts of crime and sin. Vagrancy is not regarded as a sin, but it was a great nuisance at one time and is still an offence today in certain countries. The same was at one time true of usury.

Grand larceny was not considered a crime by the mediaeval Germans. On the other hand, the conditions arising from an increase in traffic or noise may threaten society for some time before legislative action is taken. Cultural differences between countries not only influence the readiness with which old laws are abandoned and the rapidity with which new ones are made, but profoundly affect the conditions which threaten to damage society. Hoarding food is a criminal offence under recurring conditions of shortage in Greenland, but not in Europe, where these conditions do not occur.

The criminal law varies not only according to sociocultural determinants and, in particular, to those conditions which more specifically threaten a given society, but also with the power of a ruling group to impose laws, and to arrest, prosecute, and punish those who do not conform to them. In many countries, the structure of the law has, in the past, been derived mainly from a conquering, politically and economically dominant, culture, and may or may not have become assimilated to a greater or lesser extent with the original cultural framework. In Haiti, for example, the law is based, in principle, upon the Code Napoléon, but, in practice, the norms of behaviour of the indigenous population have their roots in an older traditional system, derived from their West African cultural origins. Thus, these basic cultural norms exist (though far more vitally) side by side with the official code of early nineteenth-century French origin; and in any case, the interpretation of the latter is necessarily very different in France and in Haiti. Similarly, the local interpretation of the law in Sardinia differs considerably from that of Italian law in general, though lawyers are said to be able to achieve reasonable equivalence between definitions of various crimes.

The cultural and ethical vicissitudes of the concept of crime and its punishment throughout history have been carefully documented in the works of Westermarck (1906–8, 1932, 1939), and of Fauconnet (1928). If we confine our attention to the world of today, a traveller in the West may obtain a superficial impression that there is substantial identity between the definitions of crime in different countries. It is useful, therefore, to give specific instances of the wide divergences which in fact exist.

The widest variations, though not perhaps the most important in the total field of criminal activity, occur in relation to behaviour that has the most fundamental psychological significance to man and was originally of the greatest importance to survival – namely, in matters of life and death (murder, infanticide, suicide, and other acts of violence) and sexual behaviour (marriage, promiscuity, abortion, contraception, aberrant and unproductive sexual activities). These are the aspects of behaviour which religious movements have been most concerned to control, and the definition of crime is usually related to the religious history of a culture. Property crimes, which account for about 90 per cent of what is dealt with as crime today in Western countries, have perhaps in other parts of the world more often been the concern of the conqueror and colonizer who were interested in economic exploitation, and this definition of these offences may have owed much to the historical processes of conquest and liberation.

There is widespread agreement among legislators today that the definition of heterosexual criminal behaviour is best confined to deviant behaviour that either involves the use of force or the corruption of minors, or offends against public decency. But the law and practice of many societies do not reflect these principles. In the United States, especially – no doubt because the original settlers were often members of dissident religious sects who, as well as having a strong Puritan and fundamentalist tradition, were later too busy exploring a new continent to undergo the European process of purging the criminal law of ecclesiastical concepts – adultery, fornication, and all homosexual acts are crimes in nearly every State; and, in some, masturbation or even sexual intercourse between husband and wife in any but the most conventional manner are crimes. Such acts are not, of course, commonly prosecuted as crimes but the very existence of the law makes it difficult to resist sudden public pressure for its enforcement. Women are occasionally sent to prison for adultery. Kinsey (1948) commented upon the statute which made the encouragement of self-masturbation an offence punishable as sodomy (Indiana Acts 1905, chapter 160, S. 473): 'Under a literal interpretation of this law, it is possible that a teacher . . . physician or other person who published the scientifically determinable fact that masturbation does no physical harm might be prosecuted for encouraging some person to "commit masturbation". There have been penal commitments of adults who have given sex instruction to minors, and there are evidently some courts who are inclined to interpret all sex instruction as a contribution
8

to the delinquency of minors.' In other instances, police activity in relation to courting couples or teenage promiscuity is subtly influenced by the fact that such behaviour is illegal in itself, apart from any element of offence to public decency.

Few forms of sexual behaviour have led to such anxious deliberation, or difficulties in definition, as *prostitution*. Three forms of legislative action have been adopted by various countries (and occasionally by the same country at different times) in deciding whether prostitution is a crime and, if so, under what circumstances (Mancini, 1962; Sicot, 1964).

The first, or *prohibitionist* policy, declares prostitution to be a crime at all times, and seeks to suppress it, and the trades which support it, by fines and imprisonment. This is the policy, for example, of the U.S.A., the U.S.S.R., Hungary, the Scandinavian countries, Pakistan, the Chinese Republic, some Swiss Cantons, Greenland, Iran, and elsewhere. In the U.S.A. this has led to a good deal of 'organization', the call-girl system and other devices, since the prostitute and her client are both breaking the law. In the U.S.S.R. suppression has been more successful because of close social control imposed through restriction on the transfer of capital, on which alone the white-slave traffic can flourish, and through additional devices such as publishing the names of arrested clients on a public notice-board.

The second method, of *controlled* prostitution, is based on the view that prostitution cannot be stopped but must be kept under observation and control by confining it to brothels or *maisons tolérées*, and by requiring prostitutes to register themselves and submit to periodical medical examination. This is undoubtedly the method most favoured by the clients themselves (Gibbens & Silberman, 1960), who prefer a simple and unambiguous system, and cherish the illusion that compulsory inspection reduces venereal disease. It is also the method preferred by the landlords and organizers of prostitution, since it permits the maximum financial exploitation. In the words of the French lawyer M. Mancini (1962): 'The Minister of Health, André Sellier, could write before the last war, "When I left the Government, the Friendly Society of Furnished Hotel Owners in France and the Colonies* announced that it had obtained my dismissal, thanks to powerful help at the head of the political

* The trade union of landlords of tolerated houses.

9

party to which I belonged".' The 'control' system has been under heavy attack for several decades as unjust, inhuman, inefficient, and because it implies state approval of something which it is felt should be condemned; but it exists in many countries such as Argentina, Greece, and Spain, which found themselves unable to sign the United Nations' Convention of 1949, which aimed at its abolition, and it still exists covertly in many other countries. Portugal adopts the interesting compromise of prohibiting new brothels and refusing to register new prostitutes, while continuing to licence or register those already in existence!

The abolitionist system, recommended by the United Nations' Convention of 1949 on the suppression of the trade in human beings, and accepted by most nations of the world, does not regard prostitution in itself as an offence, but demands the closing of brothels, the cessation of all registration of prostitutes, and the prosecution of those who exploit prostitutes.

France herself has shown the most agonized search for a solution in which the problems of definition were explored almost *ad absurdum*. Before 1946 soliciting was permitted at certain times and places; but, in that year, soliciting 'by gestures, words, writing or any other means' was prohibited on pain of imprisonment of up to five years. The prostitutes stood still, and no prosecutions succeeded. The police replied with a decree which defined zones where even standing and walking 'in a provocative way' were an offence; at the same time, penalties were reduced to a small fine. 'We are now at liberty to take action against prostitutes who, although not soliciting, are, by their very presence, an invitation to debauchery . . . we have defined this sort of passive soliciting.' The courts, however, decided that 'the attitude of provocation . . . was probably based on the opinions of the man in the street, . . . but the penal law cannot base itself on the intuitive method'. The problem remained. Meanwhile, France signed the United Nations' Convention in 1949 but was unable to ratify it until 1960, because, with a large army in Algeria, it was found impossible to close the brothels. Since then, severe penalties have been imposed upon those who exploit prostitutes (Mancini, 1962).

In all countries, however, when there are large movements of single men or congregations of soldiers, methods of control return covertly or overtly. Although Western Germany is an abolitionist

10

country, in both theory and practice, the city of Hamburg (Sicot, 1964) saw such an increase in public prostitution that a section of the ruined city had to be wired off. The street of 'closed' brothels, which was famous in pre-abolitionist days, had to be re-opened, but with new regulations designed to assure the freedom of the inmates from exploitation. In England, the Street Offences Act of 1959 increased the penalties for soliciting in public (cf. also Home Office, 1957).

International legislation on prostitution bears witness to the doubts which afflict societies in their desire to control many kinds of sexual behaviour. Complete suppression cannot be achieved by criminal legislation, and if laws can be applied only sporadically, they may give rise to worse evils in the form of corruption and exploitation. The aim of abolitionist legislation is to prevent the exploitation of prostitutes and to suppress the abduction and coercion accompanying the white-slave traffic, which still flourishes between France, North Africa, and South America, and in parts of the Near East.

Legislation with regard to *abortion* is apt to be interpreted in a similar way. There may be little attempt to suppress illegal abortion as such, but those who regularly practice abortion for gain are liable to incur the severity of the law.

Homosexuality provides another example of a form of behaviour which many cultures and religions have looked upon with considerable moral indifference, but which has been morally stigmatized and legally condemned with the utmost severity by Judaism and (by derivation) Christianity, and also by Zoroastrianism. In each of these religions, homosexuality was condemned particularly as a foreign cult and a practice of infidels and heretics (Westermarck, 1906–8).

According to the Zoroastrian books, there is no atonement for this 'unnatural sin', which is punished with death in this world and with torments in the next. Indeed, it is regarded as a more heinous sin than the slaying of a righteous man. 'There is no worse sin than this in the good religion. . . . It is not proper to kill any person without the authority of high-priests and kings, except on account of committing or permitting unnatural intercourse' (*Sad Dar*, ix, 2 sqq.) (Westermarck, 1906–8).

As Westermarck (1932) states, 'The early Christians' horror of sodomy has exercised a profounder and more lasting influence upon

11

moral opinion and law than their condemnation of any other form of irregular sex behaviour.' This attitude was determined by ancient Hebrew ideas (cf. Exodus, xxii, 19; Leviticus, xviii, 22–30, and xx, 13–16). 'Unnatural sin was the sin of a people which was not the Lord's people, the Canaanites, who thereby polluted their land. . . . We know that sodomy entered as an element in their religion: besides female temple prostitutes there were male prostitutes . . . attached to their temples. . . .'

'In no other point of morals was the contrast between the teachings of Christianity and the habits and opinions of the world over which it spread more radical than in their attitude towards homosexuality.' However, in eighteenth-century Europe, the influence of rationalism (and consequent anti-clericalism) brought about a change in the attitude towards homosexual behaviour.

The French Code pénal of 1810 reflected this change of outlook and replaced the earlier legislation. According to the new codified law, homosexual practices in private, between consenting adults, were no longer an offence; they were treated as a crime only when they implied an outrage on public decency, violence or absence of consent, or when one of the parties was under age or unable to give valid consent (Code pénal, art. 330 sqq.). This also became the basis of new legislation in many other countries (especially in Latin countries in Europe and America). In certain countries, such as Germany, Great Britain, and the United States, the older type of law, based on the rigid, repressive traditional attitudes, has in effect persisted to this day.

Hirschfeld's (1914) comprehensive survey of the law on homosexual offences throughout the world provides a most interesting illustration of comparative cultural and legal attitudes and traditions in this respect.

In England there have been signs of a change in the climate of opinion. The Wolfenden Committee (Home Office, 1957) made a recommendation that 'homosexual behaviour between consenting adults in private be no longer a criminal offence', which would bring English law into line with the long extant provisions of French law. This view was supported by the Church of England Moral Welfare Council (Church Information Board, 1956). Legislation to give effect to this recommendation has, however, been postponed; it is not clear where the main source of opposition to this reform lies.

The foregoing statements refer to homosexual practices between men. There is, however, an interesting difference in the relative importance attached to similar activities in the two sexes. Although in fact homosexuality in women has been, and is, widespread in all parts of the world and in many different cultures, there is no doubt that, in general, it has attracted little attention from an ethical or legal point of view: 'for the most part men seem to have been indifferent towards it; while it has been made a crime . . . in men, it has usually been considered as no offence at all in women' (Ellis, 1936). As Bailey (1955) says: 'The Lesbian's practices . . . do not imply any lowering of her personal or sexual status, and can be ignored by a society which is still in some respects fundamentally androcentric. To "corrupt" a younger girl by initiating her into the pleasures of tribadism is thought trivial compared with the "corruption" of a youth by "making a woman of him", or inciting him to inflict such a degradation upon a fellow man.'

Female homosexuality was not mentioned in the Old Testament, and, therefore, did not become incorporated in the law of most Western Christian countries. It is not an offence in English or German law – both of which treat male homosexuality with great severity. An attempt, many years ago, to extend German law in this respect failed; but Austria is one of the few countries which has long retained legislation against female homosexuality.

Kinsey (1948) observes that 'Anglo-American sex laws are a codification of the sexual mores of the better-educated portion of the population. . . . Their maintenance and defence lie chiefly in the hands of the state legislators and judges who, for the most part, come from better-educated levels. . . . However, the enforcement of the law is placed largely in the hands of police officials who come largely from grade school and high school segments of the population. For that reason, the laws against non-marital intercourse are rarely and only capriciously enforced, and then most often when upper-level individuals demand such police action.'

Crimes of violence form a second important group of offences in which there are very wide cultural and national differences in definition. One might suppose that the cardinal crime of mankind – murder – would be very similarly defined in all cultures. In practice, the variations in definition of types of homicide are large enough to make any comparison between countries very difficult. Even when

13

definitions are quite similar in law, cultural attitudes to homicide may lead to very different practice in reporting, detection, and punishment.

In general, homicide is especially prevalent in countries nearest to the equator. In Mexico, it is one of the commonest causes of death, far exceeding the local mortality rate from most epidemic diseases, and the other Latin-American countries also show a generally high rate of homicide. In Ceylon, similarly, crimes of violence are very frequent. In contrast, the homicide rates are low in Northern European, including Scandinavian, countries – with the sole exception of Finland, where the practice of carrying a knife leads to a high rate of homicide.

Indeed, cultural habits in carrying weapons profoundly affect the manner in which murder (whether of 'first' or 'second degree') and manslaughter are defined. A drunken quarrel between men carrying firearms or knives often leads to death. However impulsive the act may be, it must be assumed that death or serious injury was intended; fights with fists and boots frequently do not lead to any-one's death; should this occur, it is liable to be classed as manslaughter. Homicide by the police in countries where they are armed is also relatively frequent.

Much more fundamental attitudes to life and death, however, are involved. In some circumstances, homicide is regarded as justifiable by a culture, even when legally forbidden. In many countries of the Arab world and the Mediterranean region, or indeed until recently in some Southern States of the U.S.A. (Brearly, 1932), if a girl is seduced, either she or her seducer must die, unless a 'shotgun' marriage can be arranged. In one Arab country, a boy of fourteen was recently deputed by a family conclave to kill his sister when she brought shame on the family; he carried this out as a matter of honour in the knowledge that it was a culturally approved act. At the Cambridge Conference on prostitution in 1960, Madame Terenzio mentioned the case of a Greek girl who became pregnant in 1959. The family decided that she must drown herself. Her brother accompanied her and, when she hesitated, held her head under the water (Sicot, 1964). The extent to which homicidal family feuds may culturally be regarded as justifiable will be discussed later.

One of the earliest significant criminological observations, by Lacassagne (1886), was that in most countries the frequency of homicide varies inversely with that of suicide. In Northern European countries, especially in Denmark and Sweden, there is a high rate of suicide, whereas the prevalence of homicide is low. In most predominantly Roman Catholic countries, homicide is relatively common, whereas suicide is rare, possibly because of the knowledge that, in this religion, he who commits suicide will die unabsolved and in mortal sin. This is, however, in general equally true of the murderer, in the same countries – a fact which might perhaps suggest that local attitudes to suicide and homicide are dependent rather on deeply-rooted *cultural* influences* than on superimposed, and frequently none too clearly apprehended, Christian sectarian principles, however sincerely held, and irrespective of the individual's possible fear of eternal damnation. Indeed, it is interesting to note that, in the Middle Ages, one of the German states abolished the death penalty for murder, because it became a popular method for those wishing to commit suicide to kill some helpless defective or cripple, and subsequently to confess their crime, in the certainty that they themselves would, in consequence, be put to death. In England, nearly one-third of murderers commit suicide immediately after the crime, and many murders are 'extended' suicides, the offender killing his family as a prelude to making an attempt, sometimes unsuccessfully, on his own life. This type of suicide-murder appears to be rare in the United States: thus, in 1950, the chief pathologist of Essex County, New Jersey, where homicide is very prevalent, was able to recall only one case of murder followed by suicide in his extensive experience.

Suicide (Church Information Office, 1959; Rose, H. J., 1921; Westermarck, 1906–8; 1939) itself may not be defined as a crime. Although the earliest Patristic writings still allowed, or even approved of, suicide in certain cases, the Christian Church came to accept the uncompromising doctrine of Augustine (*De Civitate Dei*, i, 16 sqq.), which interpreted the sixth commandment as including 'self-murder', in whatever circumstances. Indeed, the influence of the traditional Christian ethic persisted for so long in English law that it was not until 1961 that, under the new Suicide Act, suicide and attempted suicide ceased to be criminal offences.

* On various cultural aspects of homicide and especially suicide, cf., e.g., the works of Bohannan (1960), Iga (1961), Sainsbury (1955), Yap (1958), and Urban (1962).

As a consequence of the former English law, the custom became widely prevalent, if not indeed universal, of presuming (whether for humanitarian or for hypocritical reasons) that in cases of suicide 'the balance of mind was disturbed' – perjury, as Bentham (1838) said, being the penance which prevented an outrage of humanity.

Another area in which legislation is apt to show great variation and ambivalence is in relation to *drugs and intoxicants*. All cultures at all times seem to have made use of whatever intoxicants came to hand, and some have shown a prevailing and almost compulsive need for them, as well as ingenuity in searching for them.* Legislation has oscillated between close control of their distribution and prohibition, on the one hand, and restriction of the possible outlets for their financial exploitation, or containment of their abuse, on the other. As with prostitution, excessively restrictive legislation has tended to give rise to abuses (such as 'bootlegging' and illicit drug-traffic), which are possibly more obnoxious than the original abuse. These examples also illustrate the quantitative aspect of the need for legislation – that laws are made only when a social problem has reached certain dimensions. More recent examples are provided by the increasing trend to control the consumption of alcohol by motorists, or that of amphetamine stimulants by teenagers.

It would be difficult to attempt to delineate the great range of factors – physiological, psychological, and cultural, sometimes general and sometimes very specific – which determine the concept of 'intoxication'. As De Quincey (1856) observed, 'some people have maintained, in my hearing, that they had been drunk upon green tea; and a medical student in London, for whose knowledge in his profession I have reason to feel great respect, assured me . . . that a patient, in recovering from an illness, had got drunk on a beef-steak'. In recent research (Connell, 1964) upon the effects of drug addiction, it was found necessary to differentiate 'addicts' who experience the effect of a drug even when given an inactive tablet of similar appearance, from those who need the drug itself in order to feel the effect.

Legislation has tended to concentrate upon control rather than

* There is a vast literature on the social and cultural aspects of the use of intoxicating drugs and alcohol, drinking patterns, etc. Reference may, however, here be made to a few valuable general works on this subject, i.e. those by Chafetz & Demone (1962); Chein *et al.* (1964); Félice (1936); Hartwich (1911); Jellinek (1960); Lewin (1931); and Pittman & Snyder (1962).

prohibition of consumption, and upon the suppression of the illegal traffic in drugs. When it was suggested that barbiturates should be prohibited because many people used them for suicidal purposes, the well-known physician, Sir Robert Hutchison (1934), observed that the logical first step should be to prohibit the sale of gas ovens. An example of man's ingenuity in discovering intoxicating drugs, even in the most remote and barren areas, is provided by the many Siberian tribes who learnt to use the dried fungus, *Amanita muscaria*, for this purpose (Lewin, 1931; Ramsbottom, 1923). In 1870, traders who bartered the fungus for furs were liable to prosecution in Russian law, but it was recorded that, in the tribes themselves, 'fungus intoxication enters into religious ceremonies and apparently is regarded as being sufficient to account for any crime and to ensure immunity from retribution' (Ramsbottom, 1923).

Nowadays, the rapid development of new drugs makes it increasingly difficult for legislative control to keep pace with their potential dangers. In post-war Japan, there was a widespread and increasing use, on the part of adolescents, of a stimulant drug, 'philopon', whose action was similar to that of the amphetamines, which, when used in excessive doses, frequently give rise to acute paranoid psychotic reactions. In a large series of cases, 40 per cent had committed some violent crime, which seemed directly related to their addiction. This drug addiction was at its height in 1954, when it was estimated that there might be 1–1·5 million of such addicts in Japan. With subsequent prohibition of its manufacture, and strict legislative controls, introduced in 1954 and (as it proved necessary) reinforced in 1955, the use of this drug has almost disappeared, but adolescents in Japan are now reported to be taking excessive quantities of barbiturate sedatives (De Vos & Mizushima, 1960; 1962; Naka, 1956). Similar legislation was introduced in England in 1964, in an attempt to control the black-market in amphetamines ('purple hearts'), especially among teenagers (*Brit. med. J.*, 1964): this type of drug was shown (Connell, 1958) to be capable of producing temporary psychosis when taken, as was frequently the case, in large overdoses.

The effect of moderate quantities of alcohol upon motor driving skill has led to new legislation. The cultural resistance to accepting this legislation in Western countries may be compared, perhaps all too closely, with the resistance of some eastern countries to accepting the legal prohibition of the sort of homicide which is approved by the culture!

Man's resourcefulness in finding new intoxicants has continued unabated – whether in making an intoxicating drink by bubbling coal-gas through milk, as was customary for many years in the slums of the larger British cities; or, as cases are at present increasingly reported, especially among juveniles and young adults, in inhaling the fumes of petrol (gasoline) and of volatile solvents in glue, etc., and addiction to a variety of more or less exotic substances (Barker & Adams, 1963; Harms, 1962; Karlsson, 1963; Laurent, 1962; Nylander, 1963; Payne, 1963; Rosenwald & Russell, 1961; Takman, 1963; Voegele & Dietze, 1963). In France, even the dogs are said to be addicted to sniffing the exhaust of stationary cars (*Field*, 1964).

Although sex crimes and crimes of violence show the largest cultural variations in definition, since many of them are not universally defined as crime at all, they are relatively unimportant in quantitative terms. In nearly all Western cultures *crimes against property* account for the vast majority of offences (80–90 per cent), and small variations in their definitions thus have a much greater effect. These variations are in fact quite substantial: the Scandinavian countries, for example, which are culturally similar to each other in many ways, have met with considerable difficulties in their recent attempt to compare their criminal statistics (Christiansen, 1960; 1965; Fredriksson, 1962).

Theft itself may be regarded in different ways. In Greenland, as we have seen, concealment of food in times of shortage is a serious offence. For a servant to take food and drink, clothes, and garden produce for himself is regarded in many countries as part of his unwritten terms of service. In Israel this form of acquisition is permitted by ancient religious law.

In Switzerland, there have been somewhat anxious discussions about whether shoplifting from self-service stores falls within the legal definition of larceny. In England, 'borrowing' a car for joy-riding is classed as 'taking and driving away' a car, and only becomes larceny in special circumstances. The young man who commits such an offence is not charged with theft of petrol, but if he uses a public telephone without paying, he is charged with 'theft of electricity'.

Apart from differences in legal definitions, complicated as they

18

are, there are much greater variations in culturally determined attitudes to the property laws. There may be 'unwritten rules' that the servant may steal from his employer, the miner take coal, the shop assistant take sweets and cigarettes, and the factory worker take scrap metal, provided the articles are for his own personal use; but his act enters a different category, amounting to theft, if it involves re-sale or secondary gain. In societies that are exposed to natural hazards, there are also accepted 'rules'. In the lonely mountain cabins in Canada the traveller is 'entitled' to take food, fuel, and clothing for urgent use, but is under a moral obligation, very strictly adhered to, to repay in whatever way he can, to replace fuel, etc. at some later date.

In recent years there has been anxiety that in complex industrialized societies there is increasing 'stratification' of the popularly accepted ideas of honesty. Few people would steal from a private individual but many will not hesitate to steal from the Government or from large impersonal organizations. Thus, shoplifting of cheap articles from self-service stores, theft of tools or materials from the work place, failure to pay for a dog licence or extra radio licence for a motor-car radio, falsification of income-tax returns, are widespread. In many countries, public opinion would regard some honest acts as 'morally obsessional', e.g. returning an excess of food allocated in error during a period of rationing.

Such dishonesty spreads throughout all sections of the community, regardless of age, class, and social position. A large number of 'perfectly legitimate' tax evasions involve adding a signature which is in fact an act of perjury, but because they cannot possibly be detected, such acts assume in practice the character of legitimacy. The fact that a certain act 'cannot be detected', that 'it's very easy', or that 'everyone does it' – especially the last – may widely determine the public attitude.

What is important from the present point of view is that although such illegal acts are widespread, they are evaluated by public opinion, and to some extent by the courts, with different emphasis. Small persistent debts may lead to imprisonment, whereas very large ones may be dealt with in the bankruptcy courts. The failure to return relatively small sums for taxation is assumed to be accidental but the act of re-selling an article before the hire-purchase instalments are completed is more often assumed to be deliberate. One is

c   19

reminded of Bernard Shaw's aphorism, that if a man steals a loaf of bread he goes to prison, while if he steals a railroad he is likely to go to Parliament. The 'man in the street' regards certain categories of behaviour as antisocial, even though the criminal law defines some aspects as illegal and others as legal. Spencer (Grygier et al., 1965, p. 233) has provided an interesting review of this problem.

'White-collar' crime may be taken as a special example, and has some interesting features of its own (Aubert, 1956; Barnes & Teeters, 1943; Sutherland, 1940; 1941; 1945; 1949). One of the most fully documented examples is the so-called 'Incredible Electrical Conspiracy' (Smith, R. A., 1961), in which twenty-nine American companies, including some of the largest and most famous organizations, were fined a total of two million dollars in 1960, for fixing prices, rigging bids, and dividing markets in electrical equipment valued at nearly two thousand million dollars a year in contravention of the Sherman Anti-trust Act. Seven executives were sent to prison (most of them for thirty days) and fined, and twenty-nine others were given suspended prison sentences or put on probation for five years. Those fixing the prices had met in great secrecy, and it was clear that all were aware of the illegality of their action, but that they were 'torn between conscience and an approved corporate policy'. One of the accused observed, however, 'It is the only way a business can be run; it is free enterprise'; another, 'Sure, collusion was illegal, but it was not unethical.' The executives sent to prison were in the upper but not the highest grade, and were subject to intense pressure from above to improve sales and profits.

Definition of Juvenile Delinquency

All the reasons for variation in the definition of adult crime apply also to juvenile delinquency, but there is an additional and much greater complexity attaching to the concept of delinquency in children. We have seen that the definition of juvenile offences appears to have arisen from a desire to provide quite different treatment for children, and to ensure this by abandoning some adult definitions. But the roots of this differentiation go much deeper.

The most fundamental question, perhaps, is how a particular culture looks upon children, and upon human growth and development. In Germany, and perhaps in England, there is a good deal of emphasis upon original sin, that a child will not develop properly unless one 'pulls out the weeds', that to 'spare the rod is to spoil the child'. Other cultures look upon the child as essentially good, and in need of only a gentle educational bending in appropriate directions, like an espalier fruit-tree. Others still, like the Chinese, appear to be entirely permissive towards children until they reach a particular age; until then, they can do no wrong, though they receive almost continuous supervision. There is little official delinquency in the children of Chinese, and notably in those of the Chinese in the U.S.A., including Hawaii (Bovet, 1951; Hsu *et al.*, 1961; Lander, 1954; Lee, 1952); though this is not to say that they do not misbehave, and in some immigrant Chinese groups there are private courts of elders who see to it that the child does not come before the public courts (Barnes & Teeters, 1943; Sutherland & Cressey, 1955). In the more complex societies, there is an increasingly detailed conception of what is good or indeed essential for the health and well-being of children; it is considered essential, for example, that they should go to school.

There appears to be little systematic information about the development of cultures in relation to the emergence of a definition of juvenile delinquency. There may be three, or four, stages of cultural change in relation to delinquency. In the first stage, in a tribal culture, there is little or no juvenile delinquency. Criminal behaviour is defined in relation to adults. In the extended family, with grandparents, aunts, and uncles exercising close supervision and control of the children of the family group, misbehaviour is prevented or punished by the parents. The neighbours have a right to punish the child, or if this fails, to complain to the parents. In Nigeria, where such conditions obtain, the nearest policeman may be many miles away. There may be considerable collusion between the families concerned to prevent any official recognition of delinquency. Only in the gravest cases, such as murder, does a local community feel that there may be general repercussions if the offender is not reported to the authority. In lesser cases, the police would in any case follow the cultural pattern of issuing warnings and rebukes. In Laos, for example, juveniles could be dealt with only by being thrown into prison, sometimes in chains; and since no responsible adult wants to see a child subjected to this treatment, little or no delinquency is reported.

21

We may note that this is precisely the procedure adopted by middle- and upper-class parents of delinquents in Western Europe and the U.S.A. whose children are at private schools. Great efforts will be made by parents and headmasters to conceal the offence, to compensate the victim, and to persuade the police (often successfully) that justice has been achieved without recourse to the law. In this type of social setting there is very little officially recorded delinquency.

In the second stage, in which the rapidly developing countries of Africa and the East are becoming involved, juvenile thieves and the like become an increasing threat to society in general, principally, it would seem, because urbanization is destroying the cohesion of families, and migration towards rapidly growing cities is forcing increasing numbers of juveniles, cut off from their tribal and cultural roots, to fend for themselves. The police force is strengthened; convictions follow for offences that would be criminal in the adult. The inappropriateness of adult punishments becomes apparent sooner or later, and as a result a separate juvenile law is evolved. The evident needs of these deprived and displaced children soon lead to preventive definitions – of being in need of care or protection, of being a wayward minor or incorrigible, etc. This tradition can be seen in many parts of the world today. In Israel, the Arab vilages, which used to be close-knit communities whose elders maintained their own system of control without much recorded delinquency, now send many young people to the large industrial building-sites. Cut off from their families, living in lodgings in strange towns, they have neither the customary controls nor the customary means of concealing their delinquency. This state of affairs is also found in many new African cities.

It is in the third stage of development, which applies to Western Europe and the U.S.A., that definitions become indistinct. The progressive development of child care and educational services, stimulated by the study and increasing understanding of the causes of juvenile delinquency, leads more and more to a preventive approach. The age of criminal responsibility is raised to enable or force the courts to consider wider aspects of the child's behaviour than the legally defined act of theft or other behaviour that would be criminal in an adult. Magistrates in some countries prefer a delinquent child to be charged as 'in need of care', even when it could, for example, be charged with theft – to the exasperation of the criminal statistician and to the alarm of those who believe that it must be brought home to a child that it has done wrong! In effect, the state, through its educational and child care services, increasingly struggles to adopt the role of the 'good parent' or the benevolent community spirit of the African villages, and to treat and educate the maladjusted child with as little recourse to legal sanctions as possible. In many countries, the age of legal responsibility is set at 14, 15, or 16, and only modified penalties are imposed up to the age of 21 or even 23. The most advanced country in this respect appears to be the U.S.S.R., where there is said to be little or no juvenile delinquency: parents are held responsible for the behaviour of their children and, if they fail, the delinquent children receive a special education as maladjusted pupils.

This process, which many would agree to be in line with what is known or believed about the origins of delinquency and many other behaviour disorders, may be followed to a greater or lesser extent, depending among other things upon cultural attitudes to child-rearing and to the respective rights of the state and of parents.

Whether this sort of cultural development occurs or not is a matter of conjecture. If it does, there are certainly many obscure factors affecting the transition from one stage to another. There are certainly many variations in evolution, as well as cultural variations in the interpretation of similar definitions. The attitudes of different societies to child development will vary in respect of the extent to which norms of behaviour are generally accepted, and deviant conduct tolerated, and the expectations and demands imposed on children. Riesman (1950), for example, has suggested that in primitive societies which are ill-protected against the hazards and vicissitudes of unaltered natural conditions, and may therefore be presumed to have a relatively short expectation of life, the educational process is stereotyped, and there is a rapid transition from adolescence to manhood. In developing countries, where there is still much poverty but also the imminent prospect of better opportunities for prosperity and a greater life-span, the child is provided over a longer period of education with internalized general rules of conduct which can be applied to the many unforeseen circumstances which he is liable to encounter in his particular socio-cultural environment. In the developed and static society, where there is a longer expectation of life and greater physical and material security, the child may be regarded as immature for a relatively longer time, and be taught mainly to conform to the customs of those around him – to 'do as the next man does'.

It may be relevant to note that a study group on 'Mental Health in International Perspective' (W.F.M.H., 1961) recorded that 'The question of identity formation has arisen as a new theoretical interest, out of studies of the significance of the newly emerging nations, the vicissitudes of the young in such a rapidly changing world, and of the effects of the prolongation of dependence that results from the spread of universal secondary education.'

In developed countries, with a 'welfare' attitude to child mis-behaviour, 'juvenile delinquency' has many meanings. New and unfamiliar forms of adolescent behaviour, which are consequently both unexpected and alarming to many adults, may all too easily become identified by the general public with delinquency as it is legally defined. As Kvaraceus (1964) has recently stated: 'Almost every language in the world now has a phrase to single out youngsters whose behaviour or tastes are different enough to incite suspicion if not alarm. . . . But we have no right to assume that every *teddy boy* or every *blouson noir* is actively engaged in delinquency. . . . It is unjust to assume automatically that a youngster who likes rock'n'roll music or bizarre clothing is on his way to becoming a delinquent, if he is not one already. Too often the adult world has used the word "delinquent" to express anger or bewilderment at adolescent tastes.' In some cases, the existence of the law is itself a motive of delinquency, the young person being spurred on by the challenge or excitement of breaking the law. It is said that in certain parts of Germany a boy is regarded as hardly normal if he does not break the law, and in some other cultural settings he is definitely expected to do so.

Although the criminologist must concentrate primarily upon those forms of behaviour which in adults would constitute crimes, he must not lose sight of the fact that he is working on shifting and uncertain ground, and dealing with ever varying factors, subject to changing social significance and fluctuating attitudes. Whatever the definition, cultural interpretations influence every stage of the process by which the fact of delinquency is established – a complaint or report by the public concerning some delinquent act, with the eventual involvement of the police who must then take action, possibly making an arrest and securing a conviction. Among the East Indians in Mauritius, a girl may be regarded as delinquent if she talks to strangers, but it is not *officially* delinquent for a girl to be promiscuous after the age of twelve. Much may depend upon whether the objective damage to society is the main concern, or whether it is the motivation of the behaviour that is regarded as socially harmful. It has been suggested that, irrespective of the legal definition, a child might be regarded as delinquent when his antisocial conduct inflicted suffering upon others, or when his family found him difficult to control, so that he became a serious concern to the community, which then reacted punitively. All these factors are subject to different cultural interpretations.

Not surprisingly, many European countries find that the years immediately following the age of criminal responsibility constitute the peak age of juvenile delinquency. Some countries are alarmed to find, as a result of an analysis of police reports, that the peak age for such behaviour is, in fact, before the age of 'criminal responsibility', and they interpret this finding to mean that, from year to year, delinquency is occurring in ever younger age groups. However, as Gibbens (1961) observed, after a survey in several countries on behalf of the World Health Organization: 'It may be that the ages of those committing acts which come to the notice of the police as offences are in fact very similar in all countries, but that this is masked by legal definitions, and that what appears to be a trend is only a permanent feature revealed for the first time. From the psychological point of view, knowledge of the age of onset of stealing – often in early years – and of the form which maladjusted behaviour first takes and how it evolves is, of course, essential to the understanding of a child's personality, however this behaviour is legally defined.'

A United Nations Report (1960) stated: 'There has been a tendency in some countries to raise the upper age limit [for juvenile offenders] to 18 or even higher. In various parts of the world, however, this position is being reconsidered, since experience has shown that the raising of the upper age limit has not taken account either of national characteristics or of the physiological and psychological development of the individuals concerned. Thus, preventive agencies, courts, etc., rather than directing attention to juveniles, often deal with a great number of persons who can, in reality, be classified as adults.'

Gibbens (1961) observes that: 'Perhaps the most important changes affecting the statistics of prevalence are the trends in definition of delinquency. In many countries new legislation is in preparation and an explanation of present procedures is followed by an account of what will be done "when the new law is passed". These differences make it impossible to compare the statistics of various countries. . . . Yet it is safe to assume that a social movement goes on for some time before it is established in the form of law, and the effect of these changes on the apparent prevalence of delinquency, even in one country, cannot be assessed.' There are, thus, formidable difficulties and very large differences in the definition of juvenile delinquency.

Kvaraceus (1964) noted that the differences from country to country with regard to offences and penalties 'only indicate how divided the world is on who is a delinquent, who is not, and what should be done about it'. A widespread form of 'delinquency' in Cairo is the collection of cigarette butts from the street. According to a recent survey in two urban areas in India, the second most common juvenile 'offence' is vagrancy (Srivastava, 1963). In Lagos, Nigeria, a delinquent is primarily an offender against the unwritten laws of the home: defiance of the family, disrespect, and disobedience are regarded as serious offences. In Hong Kong, a few years ago, no less than 55,000 juveniles were brought before magistrates' courts: of these, over 90 per cent had committed only technical offences such as hawking without a licence (Kvaraceus, 1964). Recent changes in the law now make climbing a tree a delinquent act in metropolitan Toronto (Callagan, 1961). Fruit stealing provides an interesting example of a juvenile offence of a different order, but one that is peculiar to Israel: here the law is not basically concerned with the casual picking or 'stealing' of fruit by children (which is well-nigh universal); but, in that country, the depredations on the part of immigrant children (tacitly condoned by many parents) in the orchards and orange groves in rural areas was reaching such pro-portions as to constitute a serious threat to the national economy, and, hence, to the community at large (Reifen, 1960).

In most countries, the legal upper age limit for 'juvenile' offenders lies between 16 and 19. In the United States, it differs appreciably from State to State: e.g., in Wyoming, a boy attains legal majority at 19, while a girl is a minor till 21; in Connecticut, the upper limit is 16.

The minimum age at which a child is held responsible for his acts and brought before any kind of court also varies greatly from one country to another. Thus, it is fixed at 7 in the United States, 9 in Israel, 10 (formerly 8) in Great Britain, 12 in Greece, 13 in France and Poland, 14 in Austria, Czechoslovakia, the German Federal Republic, Italy, Norway, Switzerland, and Yugoslavia. On the other hand, in some countries, such as Belgium, there is no fixed minimum age of legal responsibility.

Some twenty-five years ago Hermann Mannheim (1940; 1942) gave a clear account of the factors which can bring about statistical variations, even when the total amount of delinquency remains constant: e.g., changes in the reporting of offences by the public, police procedure (detection, arrest, and charging of offenders), changes in the law and, consequently, in the action of the courts, and changes due to the effect of the statistics themselves. If one looks at these changes in historical perspective, one finds that an increase in the number of convictions of persons under sixteen (which is not, of course, synonymous with an increase in the number of crimes committed) was noticeable in England after the introduction of the Children Act, 1908, and, especially, the Children and Young Persons Act, 1933, for the public and the police became less reluctant to charge children with offences once adequate provision had been made for dealing separately with such cases through the juvenile courts (Mannheim, 1942; Home Office, 1934). Furthermore, in considering the statistics of 1934 for England and Wales, which showed a progressive increase in juvenile convictions, 'it must be remembered that the younger the offender the easier, as a general rule, is the detection of the offence. Consequently, the figure of persons found guilty is not an entirely reliable index for the purpose of a comparison between younger and older offenders' (Home Office, 1934).

Similar examples could be quoted from the experience of several other countries.

In the course of our recent survey of the world literature on cultural factors in delinquency, a large amount of statistical material from many different countries has been examined. From these data, however, it is all too clearly apparent that, whatever their (very uneven) relative value and significance, they have little significance from a *comparative* viewpoint. It will suffice, therefore, here to mention a very few examples to illustrate the problem under consideration.

In the International Crime Statistics 1959–60 (Interpol, 1963), it is very rightly stated: 'To be of use, comparisons of data from different countries should only be made with the relative figures. . . . We do not wish to detract from the value of the statistics, which have been difficult to draw up but, to be objective, a reservation must be made. Even the relative numbers . . . only show data concerning criminals or crimes detected. Now crime detected largely depends upon the administrative and social contacts between the people and police, economic, geographical, cultural, etc. conditions.'

Let us consider, for example, the following figures selected from the International Statistics:

Country (1960)	Population (approx.) millions	Total Juvenile Offenders detected	Offenders (all ages) per 100,000 pop.
United Arab Republic (Egypt)	25·7	39	40·8
Laos (1959)	3·0	23	43·9
Federation of Malaya	7·5	508	63·7
Ghana	6·7	189	176·8
Philippines	27·5	6,082	362·3

The many sources of variation from a comparative point of view are obvious: *Who* are 'juvenile offenders'? – What are their respective 'legal' age groups? – What is the number and the efficiency of the police, and, also, the number, nature and mode of procedure of juvenile courts or other agencies (if any)? – Who reports juvenile offenders to the police, and in what circumstances? – Finally, it is necessary to take into consideration a factor of fundamental statistical importance: What was the date of the last census on which population figures, and therefore relative estimates, are based? In view of the considerable differences in the census dates of various countries, as also in the reliability and efficiency of the methods of collecting the basic data, it cannot be doubted that even the relative figures (in the last column of the foregoing table) on which we would have to rely are, in the majority of cases, inaccurate and misleading – all the more so because of the extremely rapid increase in population – and are, therefore, useless for scientific comparative purposes. (It would obviously be unrealistic to assume that even the majority of relative statistics which are presented officially have been corrected to allow for estimated annual increases in population between each census – and, indeed, such data, whether derived from the census or from interim estimates, cannot but be extremely arbitrary in the case of a large number of countries, including some of those with the largest populations.)

The low reported rate of juvenile delinquency in Laos (with all the above reservations) 'can be explained', or so it is said, 'by the social and cultural environment of Laotian families where corporal punishment is considered more appropriate for children than legal proceedings' (Interpol, 1960). This may well be so: there are not, however, sufficient cultural data available to justify any critical or confirmatory comment in this respect.

A highly developed and industrialized Western European country such as *Switzerland* – a confederation of twenty-two cantons in which are represented four linguistic and two principal religious groups* – presents an interesting example of the appreciable local variations in dealing with juvenile delinquents which may occur even in one small country (in this instance in the respective cantonal courts).†

A recent analysis (Veillard-Cybulski, 1963) of the official data on juvenile delinquency for 1961, published by the Swiss Federal Office of Statistics, shows that, in view of the diversity of the cantonal laws on procedure and judicial organization, it is certainly no easy matter to collect statistical material on this subject for the whole of Switzerland. It is, in fact, at present impossible to establish

* German (and the Low German dialect) is spoken in sixteen (almost three-quarters) of the cantons. The predominant religious groups are almost equally divided: 53 per cent of the population are Protestants (essentially Zwinglian in German-speaking and Calvinist in French-speaking cantons), and 46 per cent Roman Catholics.

† It should be noted that the present Swiss penal code (Code pénal suisse) was first introduced at the beginning of 1942 and has (except in certain specific matters) replaced by a unified code the former, *very* divergent cantonal penal laws while, at the same time, allowing the cantonal courts some considerable latitude in the interpretation of the Federal law, as also in the sentencing and disposal of criminal cases.

statistics concerning the delinquency of children aged 6–13 years, inclusive.*

The published figures, therefore, relate to young persons aged 14–19 years, and *only* those who have been subjected to a penalty or a court order. Of these, among 'adolescents' (14–17 years), boys represent 10 per cent of total male criminality, and girls, 8·4 per cent of female criminality and 12 per cent of total juvenile delinquency; the index of criminality, related to 100,000 persons of the *same age and sex*, is 1,075 for boys, and 160 for girls. For the age group of 18–19 years this index is, respectively, 2,152 and 304; and for the 20–29 year age group, 2,008 and 264. Thus, the highest delinquency rate is among the 'young adults' (approximately twice that for 'adolescents'). Since 1959, the amount of juvenile criminality has increased by about 11 per cent for adolescent boys, and 24 per cent for girls (mainly due to thefts).

The total of reprimands, officially placed at 100, does not correspond with reality, because certain cantons refuse to enter this disciplinary sanction in the police records, or replace it by an unofficial caution.† Similar procedures, whether on the part of the court or the police, are being actively extended in many countries. For example, in the United States 'It is no exaggeration to say that half the local police forces have either special departments for dealing with juveniles, or else specially trained police officers for this task. Every year, the police deal with 1,700,000 cases involving minors, only one-quarter of which are taken to the juvenile courts' (Interpol, 1960).

In Switzerland, great differences in sentencing policy are shown by the courts of the respective cantons. In 1961, Zürich imposed detention in 214 cases; Berne (with about the same number of inhabitants) in 60; Soleure in 95; Vaud in 35; and Valais in 47. The very practical measure of the suspended sentence‡ is used fairly widely in the cantons of Zürich, Vaud, Berne, Lucerne, and Geneva.

* The Code pénal suisse establishes a distinction among 'minors', between 'children' aged 6–13 inclusive (art. 82), 'adolescents' aged 14–17 years inclusive (art. 89), and 'minors' of 18–20 years, i.e. young adults aged 18 and 19 years who are also subject to special legal provisions (art. 100).

† Cf. Code pénal suisse, art. 95, which states that the court, if of the opinion that an adolescent is guilty, *will reprimand him* or will sentence him to a fine or to detention.

‡ Cf. Code pénal suisse, arts. 96–97.

It would seem to be unknown – at least, it is not used – in Valais, Schaffhausen, and other small cantons. Special treatment is also all too seldom prescribed, although this legal provision is, of course, most particularly appropriate in the case of mental defectives, who form a large proportion of delinquents* (Veillard-Cybulski, 1963). Here, as elsewhere, there is obviously a great need for the education in mental health problems of all those who are required to deal with maladjusted and delinquent children and adolescents: i.e. judges and lawyers, police officers, probation and parole officers, etc. (World Federation for Mental Health, 1961; World Health Organization, 1961).

Spain provides a particularly interesting example of the vicissitudes of the prevalence of juvenile delinquency within a relatively few years. In recent years a number of references have been made in the literature to the relatively low rate of delinquency in Spain (Bau Carpi, 1961; Bueno Arus, 1962; Hundertmark, 1962; Interpol, 1960; Ros Jimeno, 1961). Hundertmark (1962) stated that offences by minors (i.e. under 21 years) in that country had shown a considerable decrease (40 per cent) between 1953 and 1955, and also drew attention to the general decrease in the Spanish crime rate (15 per cent) during the same period. Writing in 1961, Bau Carpi stated that, while juvenile delinquency had increased in most countries, there were a few countries, including Spain, where it had in fact decreased. Similarly, Ros Jimeno (1961) quoted statistics for juvenile delinquency per 100,000 population, for the year 1959, which showed that Spain had the lowest delinquency rate of a number of Western European countries; and he further stated that the figures for juvenile delinquency in Spain were still decreasing.

The International Crime Statistics for 1959–60 (Interpol, 1963), which have become available since the above-mentioned reports were written, show that there was an increase in the relative number of offenders of all ages (i.e. per 100,000 population) in Spain, from 80·0 in 1959 to 85·5 in 1960 (and the total number of juvenile offenders also showed a very definite increase during the same period).

---

* Cf. Code pénal suisse, arts. 85 and 92 which authorize the court to order appropriate care and treatment for children and adolescents who are suffering from a mental illness or mental deficiency, or are otherwise psychologically disabled (blind, deaf-mute, epileptic).

There can be little doubt that for a number of years following the Second World War the prevalence of juvenile delinquency remained very appreciably lower in Spain than in most, if not all, other Western European countries. However, while it is quite possible that the present Spanish delinquency rate is still substantially lower than in most other European countries, it has more recently (mid-1964) been officially stated by the Spanish authorities that juvenile delinquency has quadrupled in Spain since 1951. (The actual increase, relative to population, is not yet precisely known; Spain did not contribute to international statistics of crime in 1961–2.)

The various authors mentioned above attributed – in all probability quite correctly – the consistently low delinquency rate in Spain to strong religious and traditional educational influences, and greater stability and cohesion of family life (Bau Carpi, 1961; Ros Jimeno, 1961); and (perhaps less certainly, from a comparative point of view) to better preventive measures taken by the state (Hundertmark, 1962).

Bau Carpi (1961), however, also emphasized two additional, and surely most important, factors: the lesser degree of industrialization and urbanization – and he also very cogently remarked that the latter are productive of crime only in so far as social development fails to keep pace with them.

It would seem highly probable, therefore, that because of the greater stability of the family structure and traditional values in Spain, but in addition, because of the country's economic lag for many years as compared with other Western European countries, Spain had until recently a relatively low delinquency rate. Unfortunately, according to the latest official statement, basic patterns of delinquency are now emerging in Spain significantly similar to those which have been present for quite some years in many other 'Western' countries: car-thefts have increased tenfold during the past two years, and drug-peddling and homosexual prostitution (Viqueira Hinojosa, 1962) are also reported to be on the increase. These are, indeed, all too familiar patterns. It seems certain that these quantitative and qualitative manifestations of delinquency are directly correlated with the remarkable and rapid economic development and improved standard of living which has occurred in Spain during *the past few years*.

It is interesting to note that this situation was most accurately foreseen as early as 1959 by Sarró (1961), who stated; 'The problem of juvenile delinquency reaches very small proportions in Spain, even after careful examination of the figures; but in the light of present knowledge of the causes of juvenile delinquency, this is not surprising because family and social structures have not undergone the great changes which the advance of industrialisation has brought about in other countries. Spanish psychologists, benefiting from the experience of other nations, must see to it that the social changes which inevitably follow industrialisation do not result in an increase in delinquency.'

These are but two examples of the impact of the widespread social changes occurring throughout the world today, of which many instances will be mentioned in the present report. As Bovet (1951) observed: 'The artificial nature of the concept of delinquency varies, in particular, according to the laws in force or to the way in which they are applied, and this makes it extremely difficult to establish statistical comparisons between one country and another, and one period and another. This is a major obstacle to research and a possible source of serious error. Since there is no question of unifying the laws of all countries, it is desirable that statistics on juvenile delinquency should have uniform criteria and should give a clear and detailed picture of the various kinds of offences to which they relate. The establishment of such norms is an urgent task.'

Further reference will be made to this important topic in Chapter V. It may be noted that, in the equally complex field of psychiatry, cross-cultural research has similarly been impeded by considerable difficulties in the standardization of diagnostic definitions. This question has been critically examined by Stengel (1959), and the problems of cross-cultural research in psychiatric epidemiology have been surveyed by Reid (1960), and Lin and Standley (1962).

Finally, faced as we are with these difficulties, which are so troublesome a feature of our time, it may be wise to remind ourselves that the problems of juvenile delinquency are not confined to any one period of history:

'In prosecuting these inquiries, it was found, that Juvenile Delinquency existed in the metropolis to a very alarming extent, that a system was in action, by which these unfortunate lads were organised into gangs; that they resorted regularly to houses, where they planned their enterprises, and afterwards divided the produce of their plunder. These facts, having been made known, . . . a Society was formed, the object of which was to obtain every possible information respecting the nature and causes of the evil in question, in order to ascertain the most efficient means of removing or diminishing it . . .

'The information which has been obtained may be generalised in the following order: First, that, although the judgment which the Committee are able to form, relative to the extent of Juvenile Delinquency is very indefinite, there is reason to believe, from their enquiries, that there are some thousands of boys under seventeen years of age in the metropolis, who are daily engaged in the commission of crime. Secondly, that these boys associate with professed thieves of mature age, and with girls, who subsist by prostitution. Thirdly, that such characters frequent houses of the most infamous description, where they divide their plunder, and give loose to every vicious propensity. Fourthly, that the following appear to be the principal causes of these dreadful practices: the improper conduct of parents; the want of education; the want of suitable employment; the violation of the Sabbath, and habits of gambling in the public streets. Fifthly, that, in addition to these primary causes, there are auxiliaries which powerfully contribute to increase and perpetuate the evil. These may be traced to, and included under, the three following heads: The severity of the criminal code; the defective state of the police; the existing system of prison discipline.'*

The metropolis in question is London, and the date of the Report here quoted 1816 (Report of the Committee, etc., 1816).

Nor would there appear to have been any readily discernible change, in the course of the history of the Western world, in the problem created by the divergent attitudes and mores of adults and adolescents. Thus, in Elizabethan times:

'It was the London Council that was always viewing the youth of the city with disapproval that an older generation usually feels for a younger one. It was the opinion of the Council that every young

---

* This refers to the 'moral contagion', of which John Howard (1784) wrote: 'I make no scruple to affirm that if it were the wish and aim of magistrates to effect the destruction present and future of young delinquents, they could not devise a more effectual method, than to confine them so long in our prisons, those seats and seminaries (as they have been very properly called) of idleness and every vice.'

man should spend his time working very hard for an older one, and that any sign of independence or lack of subservience to an employer was a really serious offence. The ideal apprentice was not supposed to go to a music or dancing school . . . and the Council united with the Puritans in agreeing that nothing could be worse for the morals of an apprentice than going to the theatre. The apprentices themselves did not think so, and they flocked to the theatre. . . . As a matter of fact, the apprentices belonged as a class to one of the most privileged and intelligent groups in London. . . . They were the future businessmen of London and their only crime was their youth and the fact that they loved the theatre' (Chute, 1964).

Chapter II

SPECIAL ISSUES

SEX; AGE; SOCIAL CLASS; THE POLICE

Sex

One of the facts of fundamental importance in criminology is that, as far as arrests and convictions are concerned, women are far less commonly involved in crime than men. In most Western countries, about six boys are convicted for every girl among juveniles, and ten men for every adult woman; in other parts of the world the proportion of male offenders is even larger. This remarkable discrepancy between the sexes has to be borne in mind when considering the biological, psychiatric, and psychological causes of crime. Where any particular factor (e.g. mental illness) is fairly equally distributed between the sexes, one must account for its different effect upon criminality in the sexes.

The problem has been reviewed at length by Pollack (1950) and Walker (1965). The ratio of men to women among those cautioned for or convicted of indictable offences decreases with age. In Britain, for example, the ratio is highest at the age of 20 (9·8 to 1): in the decade 50–60, the ratio falls to one man to 2·8 women, and over the age of 60, one man to 2·1 women. Women were more often cautioned than men, without being charged with offences, were possibly more leniently treated by the courts, and were more often ordered to receive some form of mental treatment (Walker, 1965).

Women may not have sufficient physical strength and agility to feel confident in committing certain crimes, such as housebreaking and robbery. Working predominantly in the home, they do not have so much opportunity for theft as men; when they do have the opportunity, as servants or when buying food in the shops, they steal more frequently. Personality tests (Rettig & Pasamanick, 1960) reveal a relatively much higher proportion of women who express conformist views about social and ethical standards. Assaults, which are relatively frequent, are directed against other women or against children. The crimes of which women are convicted more often than

36

men, in Britain, are shoplifting, cruelty to children, brothel-keeping, and procuring abortion. In the U.S.A., homicide is proportionately commoner among women serving substantial prison sentences than among men.

It has been suggested (cf. Pollack, 1950) that many of the crimes of women are in the context of a personal relationship, and are frequently not reported to the police. The servant is often dismissed without prosecution, the client of the prostitute who steals his wallet may not care to tell the police, and the girl-friend of criminals, who may have acted as watcher or decoy, may be released by the police. Few women, even if they are, for example, professional abortionists, seem to obtain much advantage, personal or financial, from their crimes. Most societies seem to feel threatened mainly by their deviant males, and the criminal law has perhaps generally been evolved to an appreciable extent, over many centuries, to deal with this particular threat. When all these factors have been taken into consideration, however, there remain a number of unsolved questions in this respect, which are of great interest to the social psychologist and criminologist.

Young girls are just as often subjected as are boys to a very unsatisfactory home life or to outright rejection. As Adelaide Johnson (1959) observed, they appear to steal from home in childhood almost as often as boys. They are, however, less frequently involved in criminal behaviour outside the home in childhood, and tend to nurse their grievances in silence and inactivity until puberty. At this stage of development, their sexual attractiveness becomes an asset which can be turned to their advantage much more successfully than the thefts and housebreakings in which boys of similar age and background are involved, and with less risk; thus they usually appear before the courts as being beyond control, in need of care or protection, or in moral danger. However, as Lady Wootton has observed, it takes two to make a sexually promiscuous act. The boys must be behaving in a similar way, as well perhaps as indulging in housebreaking. The promiscuous behaviour common to both sexes brings only the girl before the juvenile courts; the boy's behaviour is ignored.

Although some of the differences between the sexes as regards criminal behaviour may depend upon biological factors – whose importance Margaret Mead has described as being greatly exaggerated

– it is probable that most of the differences demonstrate the social origins of a great deal of crime and the social roles assigned to the sexes. Society regards it as natural and understandable – even if forbidden – for a boy to commit adventurous crimes; some cultures regard him as not quite normal if he does not do so. One may conclude that much criminal behaviour in boys represents a somewhat excessive assertion of masculinity, of proving that they conform to their sexual role, especially if they are uncertain about the latter. 'Proving' offences, especially crimes of excitement such as stealing cars or joy-riding, are commonly committed by boys whose mothers have been the dominant force. Talcott Parsons (1947) has suggested that such boys come to feel that obedience and good behaviour are feminine qualities inculcated by their mothers, so that the assertion of masculine independence at puberty involves the notion of defiance and misbehaviour. The stronger the mother's control, the more excessive is the act of breaking it. Once the demonstration has been made, however, the object of the delinquent behaviour is attained: the prognosis of 'proving' offences is, therefore, favourable when they have served their purpose. In general, it seems that the higher the educational level, the smaller the distinction between the social roles of the sexes. Psychological tests involving sex-linked attitudes and opinions fail to discriminate between the sexes in such higher educational groups. To ask a working-class boy to wash up the dishes is unthinkable; it is only the middle-class husband who accepts this as a possible duty. Since those convicted of crime are predominantly in the lowest socio-economic groups, one would expect the largest divergence here between boys and girls. It is not clear, however, whether middle- and upper-class girls are, in fact, as often involved in crime, but escape detection.

The incidence of crime at different ages falls off more gradually in women than in men, suggesting that women involved in crime, though proportionately smaller in number, are more often mentally disturbed and are relatively more persistently criminal than men, or, conversely, that male crime is more often situational and temporary. This view tends to be supported by clinical experience with women offenders. In England, as also in the Netherlands, there is a second peak of arrests of women at the age of about 45–55. These may consist of shoplifters, or of women with young children, who take to crime in their defence.

In Dakar (Pierre, Flamand & Collomb, 1963), the distribution of offences among boys and girls in 1962 was as follows:

Offence	Girls	Boys
	%	%
Theft of goods	42	49
Theft of money	3	18
Fighting	32	9
Miscellaneous	23	24
	100	100

There was a surprising excess of reported cases of fighting among the girls, apparently as a result of the relatively greater number of complaints by parents against the assailants of their daughters. Anthropologists point out that in nearly all cultures there are far fewer established rules for fighting between girls than between boys. Among boys it arouses little general interest, and they have their elaborate rules. Among girls there is no cultural definition of what is permitted, so that minor fights are reported more frequently. On the other hand, serious assaults by girls may be thought so shameful that they are not reported at all.

There is great similarity in the relative proportion of boy and girl delinquents or criminals in different parts of the world for which we have statistics. In the U.S.A. about 5 boys to 1 girl are brought to court; among adults, about 8 men are arrested and 20 men sent to prison to 1 woman. In England the sex ratio of convictions in juveniles is about 6 to 1, and 10 to 1 in adults. In Germany, the adult sex ratio is 6 or 7 to 1, but there are fewer girls among the juveniles – between about 7 and 9 to 1. In China the proportion is 10 to 1, in Italy 14 to 1, in Denmark 10 to 1, in Australia 6 to 1 (if one includes, as in England, juveniles who are found to be in need of care or protection), and in Nigeria 7 to 1. In Mauritius, however, the proportion is 20 to 1. It has been suggested that the observed range from 5 to 1 to 20 to 1 may reflect differences in the status of women in the various cultures. In developing countries the role of girls tends to be better defined; they are more protected, less subject to educational pressure, and often more affectionately regarded. They are not required, like boys, to go out and adapt themselves to a changing world.

39

Age

The relationship between age and delinquency is, of course, one of the central problems of criminology, and an adequate discussion would require a long chapter in itself. As we saw earlier, it is profoundly affected by cultural variations in attitude to the child: what is considered 'normal' for the child and what are normal expectations for the behaviour of children. In Western societies people will say of a boy of twelve: 'After all, he is only a child.' In more primitive societies, with a shorter expectation of life and a more urgent pressure upon the young person to contribute to adult society, the attitude may be: 'After all, he is almost a man.'

The most important question relating to the age of the delinquent concerns his maturation, or the age at which delinquency comes to an end. In most countries the incidence of delinquency is highest at some time during adolescence, usually between 14 and 16, and falls away rapidly after 21 or, at most, 25. The majority of children or adolescents who appear before a court do so only once; and the majority of those who persist for a time stop their criminal behaviour, or at least are not arrested, after the age of 21 or 25. On the whole, the younger the boy at his first conviction, the greater the chances of reconviction. There is a good deal of evidence that those who persist in crime well into adult life include a somewhat excessive proportion of men who were first convicted when quite young. On the other hand, more recent studies of persistent offenders of 30 or 40 (West, 1963; Gibbens & Silberman, in press) show that a surprisingly high proportion – 40–50 per cent – have not been convicted before 17, and in many cases not before 21. There are, therefore, serious doubts about the proposition that the earlier a person commits crime, the longer he is likely to go on doing so. Sheldon and Eleanor Glueck, from a study of their massive data, reached a somewhat intermediate conclusion that delinquency 'regardless of age at the time it begins . . . runs a fairly steady and predictable course' (Glueck & Glueck, 1940). 'On the whole, if the acts of delinquency begin very early in life, they are abandoned at a relatively early stage of manhood, provided various mental abnormalities do not counteract the natural tendency to maturation. . . . If, on the other hand, the acts of delinquency begin in adolescence, the delinquent tendency seems to run its course into a later stage of adulthood, again, however, provided the natural process of maturation is not interfered with' (Glueck & Glueck, 1945). Criminological theories on the age of the offender have been extensively reviewed by Barbara Wootton (1959). She concluded, 'there has been little significant advance since Sellin'; indeed, after an extensive review of relevant material, some twenty-five years ago, Sellin (1940) came despondently to the conclusion that 'the research student who in the pursuit of an answer to the relationship of age to crime consults the reports just mentioned, is doomed to disappointment'. This, the most important of all relations to age, still remains very uncertain. If we do not know the situation in any one country, we cannot make any estimate of cultural differences in this respect.

The Topeka Conference directed its attention mainly to the age-trends in delinquency in the countries represented. In ancient times, age and the associated legal criteria, were related to the physical signs of puberty, etc; in Nigeria today, no doubt for the same reason – the absence of birth certificates – much of the doctors' time in a child guidance clinic is spent in making estimates of the age of juvenile offenders.

In European countries, the age of criminal responsibility varies widely – from 8 or 10 to 14, 15, or 16; it does not necessarily follow that the treatment provided differs widely. By special research, it is possible to consider the behaviour of children, under the age of responsibility, which would have been classed as delinquent if it had occurred in adults. Subject to the reservations which were mentioned earlier, concerning statistics of juveniles, one can make some tentative comparisons.

In Germany, England, Canada, and Japan (all heavily industrialized countries undergoing rapid technological development), there appears to be an increase in recorded delinquency in the older adolescent age group – a relatively new phenomenon.

In Germany, adult crime has remained relatively constant in the last ten years; the general increase in crime is mainly attributed to an increase in juvenile crime, especially in the age group 18–21, and to some extent in younger groups. Since these older adolescents are constantly being recruited into the adult group, which is *not* showing a steady increase in crime, it is assumed that this late adolescent delinquency is a normal developmental phase which most boys grow out of quite successfully; if so, it may be questioned whether it need be taken very seriously. It is reported in many countries that the attitude of the magistrates, and perhaps the public in general, tends to be strongly punitive towards this age group, who are thought of as 'old enough to know better, and not just children'. It is an open question whether such adolescents settle down quickly because they are forcefully resisted by society and the courts, or because they are passing through a transitory phase which will terminate regardless of the degree of repression. Both hypotheses are quite tenable, and the issue can only be solved by experimental study.

In Japan, adult crime has been steadily decreasing for the last six years, but total crime has been held constant by an increase in the age group 15–18. By special police measures and other facilities, the crime rate in this age group has, however, been stabilized in the last two years. As in other countries with a rapid increase in the number of automobiles, traffic offences by youths have increased sharply.

In Canada, the group from 16–19 has been largely responsible for the increase in crime. In 1954 this age group was responsible for 18 per cent of crime, but in 1961 this figure had risen to 30 per cent. The contribution of girls of 16–19 has also risen from 16 per cent to 19 per cent of female crime. These increases may be connected with the increase in size of the age group. In Taiwan, the increase has been in the 16–18 age group.

In England there has been a similar sharp increase in the criminal behaviour of the age group 17–21. That these countries were all involved in a world war as full combatants suggests that the trends may be due to the disruption caused by war. Apart from the aggressive ideas inculcated in children in wartime, there is the persistent nostalgia of ex-combatants who allow their children to perceive their preoccupations. This important problem was considered in detail by the Roffey Park Study Group (World Federation for Mental Health, 1961), which reported as follows:

'In 1961, there is less emphasis upon the effectiveness of particular types of child rearing practice in preventing destructive aggression. On the other hand, the argument that warfare is ineradicable because it has its roots in human aggressiveness is now opposed on the following grounds: First, that it cannot be shown historically either that warfare arises from individual destructiveness, or that it is basically derived – especially in the case of modern warfare – from the individual's willingness to engage in combat. Secondly, protective impulses directed towards the young, and towards one's country and ideals, play a very important part in the involvement of human beings in war. The problem of preventing war, therefore, resolves itself very largely into the development of social patterns which will continuingly reduce the possibility of conflict, rather than reliance, to any appreciable extent, either on different types of character formation, or upon the direction of aggressive impulses into socially constructive channels.'

In England, Wilkins (1960) made a statistical analysis of the delinquency rates of different age groups of juveniles, and concluded that the greatest 'crime-proneness' was found in those who had passed through their fifth year during the war period, 1939–45, constituting a 'delinquent generation'. The suggestion was made that the age of five or thereabouts represents the time when *social* communication is at its height, and when the standards, principles, norms, and expectations of the social group are being communicated to the child. Though emotional development may be determined in the first five years, succeeding years may profoundly influence verbal communication and the development of social concepts.

Not all countries, however, have shared in these developments. In Belgium, the lowest age groups have shown the greatest increase in delinquency, giving rise to the idea that the younger the child, the more profoundly he reacts to environmental change. In Italy, juvenile delinquency has been decreasing at the rate of 5–6 per cent per year. It is assumed that the effect of wartime disturbance has passed its peak.

In Norway, research into police records has shown that the peak age of delinquent activity is fourteen, below the age of criminal responsibility. In Denmark, the peak, at fifteen, occurs with the onset of responsibility and is not thought to antedate it. As will be seen later (pp. 130–1), the concept of a 'delinquent generation' has also been explored in Denmark (Christiansen, 1964).

One hypothesis which has been raised is that delinquency may have a similar incidence at all ages, but that boys are more easily caught at the peak ages. After early adolescence, they may become more careful and cautious. Sveri (1960) has shown that before the age of fifteen the majority of offences are committed by groups of boys; thereafter, the solitary offender begins to predominate, and this tendency increases rapidly. One of the many reasons for this change is increasing sophistication and the knowledge that one is more liable to escape detection best by committing a crime on one's own and trusting no one. Policemen, with their day-to-day practical experience, seem to regard bad luck and lack of skill as playing a large part in the incidence of detected delinquency, but criminologists regard the peak age as broadly parallel to the actual incidence of crime. Confidential interviews with recruits to the army, in countries having universal conscription, have tended to confirm that the peak ages of detected and undetected crime are roughly similar. The public and the police probably regard the misbehaviour of particular age groups, especially seventeen- and eighteen-year-olds with more alarm and exasperation than that of younger boys; this may influence arrests when there are several age groups to choose from, as may be the case in riots and other group disturbances.

Many believe that with increased mobility and industrialization, there is an increased tendency to report offences that occur in cities. It is, however, uncertain whether certain age groups are more particularly affected by these changes.

Social Class

It is widely believed that delinquents include an excessive number from the lowest socio-economic classes. The evidence for this view is, however, very slight. In a critical review, Wootton (1959) remarks, 'We thus reach the surprising conclusion that, on the definitions used by these investigators, those who find themselves in trouble with the criminal law on either side of the Atlantic are predominantly drawn from the lower social classes but, even so, we are not able to say whether, or how far, this predominance exceeds that to be expected from the proportion which these classes contribute to the non-criminal population.'

Several studies, however, indicate a modest tendency for the fathers of delinquents to be unskilled rather than semi-skilled or skilled and also, as is, for example, shown by the Gluecks (1950), for a lower proportion of fathers of delinquents to have a business of their own (3·5 per cent compared with 8·5 per cent) or to be employed as clerks, salesmen, insurance brokers, lawyers, etc. (2·4 per cent compared with 4·5 per cent).

A question that interests sociologists is whether the observed difference in social class – assuming that one accepts that there *is* a difference – is not largely or wholly accounted for by a different attitude to such middle-class delinquents by the police and other authorities. An expectation by the police that crime is to be found among the poorest classes may lead to more concentrated activity in the areas of the city where they live. By contrast, the middle-class boy is often in a protected environment, such as a boarding-school where any stealing or other delinquency is punished by the head-master rather than the courts. Even when they occur in the general community, many delinquent acts do not go beyond the stage of being reported. Parents know how to enlist the help of other community resources: the boy is taken to a child guidance clinic for advice; if necessary, he is sent to a residential school for maladjusted children. Understandably, the police may not proceed with a case which is clearly being dealt with vigorously by the family, or means are found of preventing the case being reported to them at all. Delinquents committed to reformatories are likely to include a higher proportion of lower-class boys than those brought before the courts or merely reported to the police; studies based on institutionalized boys may, therefore, be misleading. In the countries of Western Europe, with a broadly based democracy, this effect is probably less marked than in countries, such as some of the South American states, where political power is concentrated in the hands of a small oli-garchy. It would be surprising if the police were not sensitive to prosecuting the sons of their employers. The police share the general attitude of the community to social class, and are influenced, if only in borderline cases, by social pressures and prejudices. In New York, it is said to be an advantage, if arrested, to speak with an Irish brogue, since so many of the police are Irish. In Italy, the accused try to speak with a Milanese rather than a Sicilian accent!

Such social-class differences in treatment extend into the mental health field. Hollingshead and Redlich (1958) have shown that the lower-class patient with a schizophrenic psychosis may not be released at all from a State hospital, or is at least detained per-manently after the first unsuccessful attempt at rehabilitation in the community; the upper-class schizophrenic may be repeatedly discharged and re-admitted and given intensive out-patient psycho-therapy. The middle- or upper-class family can organize many social resources to help to rehabilitate the delinquent or the psychotic.

Social-class differences may explain the results of other researches. Racial differences may be due ultimately to social-class differences if, for example, the coloured population, predominantly working-class, has more delinquency than the white population, which is largely middle-class. Recent research suggests that *homogeneous* Negro communities in cities of the U.S.A. may be no more delinquent than socially comparable white populations, but that Negroes may be more delinquent in mixed sections of the city (Lander, 1954; Savitz, 1962). In Mauritius, the level of delinquency among the Chinese remains fairly constant, but has risen among the Muslims and mixed coloured population, while declining among the Indian Hindu population. In recent years, the Hindu population has achieved political ascendancy, and the mixed coloured population especially tends to feel excluded and insecure.

Social mobility from one class to another, which is nowadays perhaps more widespread because of new economic and educational opportunities, may produce stress in a family while it is relatively isolated between one social class and another. Old loyalties are thrown aside, but new ones are only partially accepted; fathers and sons may observe different standards. Social mobility leads to different expectations of behaviour, which in turn lead to variations in reporting offences. An increase in assaults may consist partly of more frequent domestic quarrels; when rehoused on a new estate, some wives may not tolerate the sort of behaviour from husbands which is common in a slum area. In a slum, local opinion discourages any reporting to the police; on a new estate, it may not be 'respectable' not to do so. A study of cases of violent cruelty to children some years ago (Gibbens & Walker, 1956) revealed a number of cases where cruelty had rather surprisingly *followed* rehousing in much better circumstances. Families whose children had run wild in slum conditions had become conspicuous: neighbours complained and dropped hints to the parents about the need for punishment. When the parents beat the children severely, the same neighbours reported them to the police!

Similarly, social-class differences and potential animosities may be inflamed by building a slum-clearance estate in the midst of a middle-class area of a city. The 'estate boys' are blamed for all the delinquency in the area, and feel the need to keep up a vendetta of provocation against their 'stuffy' neighbours.

An increase in 'middle-class' delinquency is reported especially from Belgium, Canada, and Japan. It is not clear whether this is a genuine proportionate increase, or whether it is due merely to an increase in the total middle-class population, as the result of much greater economic and educational opportunities. Clinicians from many countries have the impression that they see more delinquents who attend grammar schools or high schools, and whose parents are employed in the clerical and professional occupations; but these are the very groups that make use of psychiatric services, and it would be unwise to judge from such experience without knowing whether this sort of family is becoming more prevalent in the general community.

In England, attendance at grammar schools or in advanced educational classes was much more common among children convicted of shoplifting than among those convicted of other forms of delinquency (Gibbens & Prince, 1962). Other forms of delinquency, such as car-stealing, tend to be class-linked because the activity does not come within the range of aspiration of the lower-class youth; but as car-ownership spreads to all socio-economic groups, this difference diminishes.

Pressure to make the most of new educational openings and to rise in social class produces many tensions. The boy who makes a great deal of progress and then fails at high school for emotional reasons – a fairly frequent type of delinquent – may have detached himself conceptually from his neighbours, yet fails to attain the new status that has been placed within his reach. The use made of educational opportunities may also vary with the social class of the parents. In Nigeria, for example, where education is free but not compulsory, it was found that 27 per cent of children did not go to school at all, 29 per cent had started but later stopped attending, 18 per cent were irregular attenders, and 26 per cent went regularly to school. Profit or lack of profit from education may be expected to accelerate the great social mobility and the differentiation of contrasted strata of society. In some countries, such as Mauritius and many newly developing countries, there may be little employment available except to adults. The boy who leaves school at fourteen may have many years of relative idleness before he can expect a man's job; but the boy who is capable of higher education is fully employed on his studies or is eligible for apprenticeships. Jobs with limited scope for advancement (e.g. messenger in clubs or cafés) often bring the boy into contact with less stable sections of the population.

Lastly, one may ask whether upper-class fashions and eccentricities influence the delinquent behaviour of the lower class. The spread of mass-communication by radio, television, etc. has perhaps deprived the 'ruling classes' of much influence and substituted that of the popular idol or pop-singer. The majority of these influences on clothes, speech, and manners are probably very superficial and harmless (if extremely lucrative to industrial producers who play a large part in promoting them). But some observers think that there are undesirable fashions – highly promiscuous parties, demonstrative behaviour by pseudo-homosexuals, or drug-taking – which may spread down the social scale.

The Police and other Law-enforcement Agencies

No one plays a more important part than the police in the control of delinquency, and cultural variations in their practice and social role have the greatest significance. In many countries these are changing rapidly and sometimes produce doubts and confusion. In one city in the United States, for example, 60 per cent of juvenile cases involve warnings for delinquent tendencies (truancy, fighting, trespassing, etc.), 23 per cent involve minor offences dealt with by warnings and police supervision; and only 17 per cent involve major offences which are referred to the juvenile court. In England, the police have only recently developed the supervising and controlling role, by developing police liaison schemes in selected cities, as opposed to the role of detection and prosecution. Police in small country districts, however, traditionally exercise the controlling function, and it is perhaps the process of rapid urbanization which emphasizes the need to combat crime and delinquency.

The police are dependent upon the support of the community, and are much more sensitive to changes in public opinion than the courts or judges. In exercising a supervisory role on their own initiative, the police reflect the social attitudes of the classes from which they are recruited. Lawyers, magistrates, and judges also reflect class attitudes, but are usually recruited from the middle and

upper classes and show little class mobility or flexibility in the course
of their lives. In relation to sex and aggressive behaviour expecially,
in which the norms show marked social-class differences, lawyers and
magistrates are likely to reflect the views peculiar to their own class.
They and the police are likely to show different attitudes to minority
groups.

Increasing supervision requires closer collaboration with other
social agencies. In referring cases for psychiatric advice, for example,
the police often pick out the sexual offenders. They know that they
will have to supervise such people in the community for some time,
and are uncertain how to do so. This collaboration varies a great
deal from force to force, or even from one area to another in a city,
depending upon how particular officers perceive their social role.
Close collaboration with other agencies, e.g. medical services, can
give rise to a number of difficult ethical problems.

The police must steer a difficult path between three sets of
relationships – to the public, to the offender, and to the law agencies.
Thus, in England, 62 per cent of all offences involve motoring
behaviour: and these may concern otherwise law-abiding sections
of the community. It has been supposed that the police are in
danger of becoming unpopular if they enforce the regulations too
severely. In relation to juveniles they must adjust themselves to
popular attitudes to the child.

Unpublished studies of juveniles – offenders or otherwise – reveal
the essential ambivalence of their attitude to the police. Rebellious
attitudes to authority are apt to be symbolized by an overt hostility
to the police, yet such young people have a deep respect for the
police, and expect them to show the highest standards of behaviour.
Much depends, therefore, on the adolescent's first contact with the
police, just as the admission procedure to a hospital may colour
the patient's attitude. Rough handling or lack of human respect
quickly produces bitterness and cynicism in the delinquent. By
contrast, the adult recidivist frequently recognizes that the police
are doing their job and has no animosity against them. It is much
easier for the police to deal fairly with the adult offender than with
the adolescent who deliberately provokes hostility.

Lawyers and other agents of the court complicate relations with
the offender by having to advise him to say nothing or to impede
the process of justice. The obstruction is apt to increase the hostility

of the police towards the offender. In some countries, such as India, confessions are not admissible as evidence. In others, the examining magistrate (*juge d'instruction*) takes over the investigating and prosecuting function, allowing the police to assume a more neutral role. A high price for these procedures, however, is paid in long delays before conviction is obtained.

An interesting example of the consequences of special pressure on the police by higher authority was provided by the teenage riots in Copenhagen, which were specially investigated. The results, given below, show how a change of police policy may affect both the number of arrests and the type of juvenile arrested. Large-scale teenage riots have been rare in Denmark, but after the showing of the film *Rock around the Clock* there was an exceptional riot which lasted for no less than six days. Thousands of teenagers congregated in the main square or roamed the streets. For the first two days, the police followed a policy of 'wait and see', intervening only when it was unavoidable. On the third day, 'preventive' action was ordered: the police were instructed to intervene before trouble occurred. On the fourth day, instructions were amended: police were to adopt a permissive attitude.

Arrests

First day   (expectant)   9   Fourth day (permissive) 7
Second day (expectant) 14   Fifth day   (permissive) 0 (it rained)
Third day   (preventive) 30   Sixth day   (permissive) 3

The type of juvenile arrested was as follows:

	Previous Arrests	Nil
Third day	10	20
Other days	21	12

By contrast, in one Latin-American country, the magistrates adopt such a permissive attitude to the delinquents who come before them that the police feel there is little use in arresting and charging deliquents. They tell citizens: 'Be sure to punish any delinquent you catch before we arrive, because you may be sure that after we have made the arrest, no further action will be taken.'

These considerations apply to some extent in most European countries. In other parts of the world, however, the image of the police may be very different. In underdeveloped countries, the police may be rarely seen; occasionally, they may be rough or corruptible; and they may be regarded with suspicion. Small communities may keep information from them, refuse to co-operate in inquiries, or give evidence against them. In some newly independent countries, the police have to overcome hostility and suspicion due to their former status as representatives of alien domination.

There are, of course, many varieties of police organization. Several countries have two forms of police – para-military national police as well as a local police system, and public attitudes towards the two forces differ. The carabinieri in Italy, and rather similar forces in some Mediterranean and South American countries, have a higher standard of education, training, and morale, and greater discretion in settling disputes or making final decisions. They usually operate alone in country districts, and may then adopt a highly respected paternal role. There were instances in the Second World War when carabinieri identified themselves so closely with their communities that they were shot as hostages on behalf of their folk. The Royal Canadian Mounted Police also have a tradition of independent action. Police of this kind are feared by the serious offender but may be consulted by the first offender.

Judges and magistrates vary in their sentencing policy, both for personal and for cultural reasons. These variations have been the subject of many recent studies (Hood, 1962) in individual countries, but there are probably great variations between one country and another in the general standard adopted and the degree of consistency with which it is applied. In one country, as we saw, the magistrates take such a lenient view of juvenile delinquency that the police feel it is useless to make arrests. Many police forces probably feel that delinquents are not dealt with severely enough. Those countries which appoint magistrates or judges for life must surely have some traditional confidence that certain standards will be maintained. Magistrates in other countries, who are subject to fairly frequent re-election, are perhaps more sensitive to public opinion. The machinery of justice, especially the extent to which cases are subject to appeal, affects uniformity of practice. In Norway, for example, *all* decisions of the juvenile tribunals are subject to automatic review by the higher court; this must surely make for uniformity of sentence.

Chapter III

SUBCULTURES: SOCIAL THEORY

The word 'subculture' has moved into general currency in the last twenty years, not only among sociologists. It is even possible for the psychiatrist to speak of the 'subcultural type' of delinquent with a good deal of consensus among his colleagues as to what he means by this term. Kluckhohn (1964) quotes the definition by Gordon (1947): '. . . a subdivision of a national culture, composed of a combination of factorable situations such as class status, ethnic background, regional and rural or urban residence, and religious affiliation, but forming in their combination a functioning unity which has an integrated impact on the participating individual.' This is the sense in which it is used here. To the cultural anthropologist, who has a proprietary right to the term, it may have a different meaning, implying a common attitude to certain fundamental human functions such as traditions about property, marriage, and child-rearing. In many cases he would prefer 'culture-variant' to 'subculture'. Thus, although the layman may speak of 'Latin-American culture', he can be assured that there is no such thing in any anthropological sense; there are several distinct Latin-American cultures, each of which may have culture-variants.

The general discussion of subcultures at the Topeka Conference presupposed a familiarity with the main lines of development in social theory in relation to delinquency. These cannot here be described in detail, but it may be helpful to give a brief outline of the main developments. Many of these theories have originated in the U.S.A. They have been excellently reviewed by Wolfgang, Savitz, and Johnston (1962), and a critical and thoughtful assessment has recently been made by Clinard (1962) – cf. also Merton & Nisbet (1963). Valuable as they are, one must remember the special relevance of these theoretical concepts to the social conditions upon which they were based, and also endorse the comment of Wolfgang and his co-editors, 'that increasingly from Shaw and McKay to the present time, decreasing amounts of data are presented, and increasingly the emphasis is on the presentation of

52

logic-tight theories which may or may not be ultimately valid'.

The nineteenth-century French criminologist, Lacassagne (1886) was among the first to emphasize the importance of the social environment. Crime, he considered, only flourished in a social medium specifically appropriate to its development: 'Societies have the criminals they deserve.'

Emile Durkheim may justly be regarded not only as a pioneer of French sociology, but also as one of the founders of criminal sociology, whose work has only recently received the attention it deserves. He boldly stated (1895) that crime is 'an integral part of all healthy societies', and is 'bound up with the fundamental condition of all social life, and by that very fact it is useful, because these conditions of which it is a part are themselves indispensable to the normal evolution of morality and law'. If one could imagine 'a society of saints, a perfect cloister of exemplary individuals', the most serious deviations, which we might regard only as minor faults, would still be defined as serious infringements and would create the same scandal as those acts which we call major crime today. In such an orderly and homogeneous society, the inevitable processes of biological variation would ensure that some deviant conduct occurred which was regarded as criminal. Any evolution or positive change in a society could not occur without negative or unwanted variations. Most important, perhaps, Durkheim also described, in his work Le Suicide (1897), the concept of 'anomie' – 'l'état de dérèglement ou d'anomie', which 'results from man's activity lacking regulation'. Bierstedt (1964) quotes its definition by MacIver (1950) as 'the fulfilment of the process of desocialization, the retreat of the individual into his own ego, the sceptical rejection of all social bonds'; it 'signifies the state of mind of one who has been pulled up from his moral roots, who has no longer any standards but only disconnected urges, who has no longer any sense of continuity, of folk, of obligation'.

The rise of a more scientific sociology of crime began only some four decades ago, when the first textbook reflecting this orientation was published by Professor E. H. Sutherland (1924). Since then, according to Sellin (1938), 'a dozen or more similar texts have appeared, all but one written by sociologists, all of whom, true to a traditional view of the scope of criminology, have felt compelled to present, examine and criticize all kinds of criminological research, including that emanating from sciences of which they usually have had only limited basic knowledge'. Sellin himself, as this quotation implies, has never been inclined to overstate the claims of sociology. 'Man,' he insists, 'is born into a culture . . . he absorbs and adapts ideas . . . which embody *meanings* attached to customs, beliefs, artefacts, and his own relationships to his fellow men and to social institutions. Looked upon as discrete units, these ideas may be regarded as *cultural elements* which fit into patterns or configurations of ideas. . . . Embodied in the mind they become *personality elements*, and the sum total of all such elements may be conveniently called *personality*, as distinguished from the person's biological individuality or his inherited and acquired morphological and physiological traits. Personality then rests upon a biological foundation, which is of the greatest importance in the formation of personality. The biological make-up of an individual fixes limits to personality development, determines the character of the receptive and adaptive processes which transform cultural elements into personality elements, and influences the latter's experiences in social activity.' If it is objected by psychologists that 'personality is more than "the subjective side of culture" ' (Allport, 1937) and involves various psycho-physical systems, the sociologists must reply that they are not psychologists or biologists, and are entitled to place 'upon their enquiries the limitations imposed by their science' (Sellin, 1938). This quotation, in the editors' view, perhaps sums up the common ground upon which the many disciplines represented at the Topeka Conference were able to conduct their discussion.

Sutherland's own contribution (Sutherland & Cressey, 1955), subsequently defended and perhaps extended by Cressey, was to evolve the theory of 'differential association'. 'Criminal behaviour is learned in interaction with persons in a pattern of communication.' 'A person becomes delinquent because of an excess of definitions favourable to violation of law over definitions unfavourable to violation of law.' 'When persons become criminals, they do so because of contacts with criminal behaviour patterns and also because of isolation from anti-criminal patterns.' The two sides of the latter statement must be especially noted.

In his vigorous defence and detailed elaboration of this theory, Cressey (1960) emphasizes that it is not limited merely to ideas of 'bad companions' or the underworld associates of the professional criminal; nor are criminal patterns learnt necessarily or only from criminals. Sutherland himself went on to admit that 'the process of learning criminal and anti-criminal patterns involves all the mechanisms that are involved in any other learning'. Later on we shall return to the question of whether this is not, as Cressey suggests, the most generally valid theory of crime. One may, however, ask whether any *general* theory for such a vast and heterogeneous range of behaviour as crime can be more incisive than a platitude, or can have any heuristic value. The theory does, however, appear to encompass subsequent social theories and indeed most of what psychiatrists or psychologists believe about crime (cf. Cressey, 1964).

Sellin's (1938) own special contribution was in his description of the 'culture-conflict' element in crime, of which many examples will be provided below. When cultures with quite different norms of conduct meet in contiguous areas, or when members of one culture migrate to another, or when alien laws are imposed by conquering or colonizing powers, offences of this kind arise for obvious reasons. The majority of inhabitants of Mexico or certain West Indian islands may break the alien and imposed laws regulating marriage. In several Mediterranean cultures it is expected that a girl who is seduced, and dishonours the family, will be killed by father or brother as a matter of duty, however painful. In some cases of this kind there is no mental conflict, only surprise that the behaviour is classed as criminal. In other cases, there is mental conflict, the clash of antagonistic norms of conduct derived from divergent cultures and incorporated in the personality. Within a culture, rapidly changing subcultures, or first- and second-generation immigrants, may suffer such conflicts of norms which produce criminal behaviour. Sellin at the same time draws attention to the need to study criminal behaviour in terms of the extent to which norms have been internalized by individuals as elements of the personality. Clearly, there is a problem, in culture conflict, of the tenacity with which old norms are maintained, even if no longer appropriate (cf. Wirth, 1931).

In Chicago, where mass immigration of Italians, Poles, and other nationalities took place in waves, and where, as a result partly of bootlegging and partly of economic difficulties, an underworld of successful criminals became a sight familiar to all, Shaw and McKay (1942) were able to demonstrate that certain sections of the city produced a high rate of delinquency from one generation to another as a matter of direct cultural transmission. Boys in such areas might be presented with an evenly balanced choice of delinquent or non-delinquent behaviour, in which friendship, loyalty, status, and opportunity might be on the side of delinquency. Such boys are not necessarily disorganized, maladjusted, or antisocial within the limits of their social world and in terms of its norms and expectations. Such delinquents, who have been termed 'pseudosocial' (Jenkins, 1949), or 'well-trained to antisocial standards' (Scott, 1960b), are to be found in all large cities of the Western world, no doubt, though they constitute perhaps only 5–10 per cent of institutionalized delinquents (Jenkins, 1949).

Merton (1938), developing Durkheim's view of anomie, pointed out that there are two elements in the social and cultural structure which can be considered separately, although they tend to merge imperceptibly in concrete situations. There are, first, culturally defined goals, purposes, and interests which draw impulse from biological drives, but are not determined by them. They provide a frame of reference for the aspirations of the individual, such as choice of occupation. On the other hand, 'the social structure defines, regulates and controls the acceptable means of achieving these goals', with moral and institutional regulation of permissible and required procedures for attaining them. Cultures or parts of cultures may emphasize one or other side of the balance. If too much emphasis is placed on the end rather than the means, upon winning the match rather than playing the game, then the play becomes 'dirty'. On the other hand, the caricature of the bureaucrat is of a man whose goal of efficient service is so far attenuated that the institutional norm of 'going through the proper channels' becomes predominant. And perhaps religious institutions, whose goal of perfection is far removed from immediate attainment, emphasize, as in monasteries, a relatively rigid social structure. In the conformist majority of social institutions, goals and means are balanced so that the individual obtains adequate satisfaction. An exaggerated and spontaneous ambition, *or* severe lack of opportunity, do not respectively provide a sufficient explanation of delinquency. 'It is only when a system of cultural values extols, virtually above all else, certain *common* symbols of success *for the population at large*, while its social structure rigorously restricts or completely eliminates access to approved modes of acquiring these symbols *for a consider-*

56

able part of the same population, that antisocial behaviour ensues on a considerable scale.' 'The American stress on pecuniary success and ambitiousness for all thus invites exaggerated anxieties, hostilities, neuroses and antisocial behaviour' (Merton, 1938). This analysis helps to explain the lack of any regular relation between poverty and crime. Later on, we shall have to consider what effect repeated massive immigration may have had upon the development of this goal of pecuniary success, the fact that among many norms this survives as common to all, and to what extent a similar social development may be overtaking many other rapidly developing countries of the world.

Cohen (1955) has discussed the subculture of delinquents with a realistic sense of the great variety of their behaviour, and the differences to be seen between motivating factors which centre upon the commission of the act itself (cf. Tiebout & Kirkpatrick, 1932). 'There is no accounting in rational and utilitarian terms for the effort expended and the danger run in stealing things which are often discarded, destroyed or casually given away. . . . What we see when we look at the delinquent subcultures . . . is that it is *non-utilitarian, malicious* and *negativistic.* It is defined by its "negative polarity" to the norms of respectable society. That is, the delinquent subculture takes its norms from the larger culture, but turns them upside down. The delinquent's conduct is right by the standards of his subculture, precisely *because* it is wrong by the norms of the larger culture' (Cohen, 1955). As Shaw and MacKay (1942) had observed, 'the standards of these groups may represent a complete reversal of the standards and norms of conventional society'.

Studies in Chicago by Shaw and McKay were continued by Kobrin (1951). It has often been stressed that even in heavily delinquent areas the majority of boys are not convicted of delinquency or the subject of police reports. From a careful analysis of detailed records, he showed that, not counting any boy more than once, some 66 per cent of the relevant juvenile population were reported to the police at some time during the years when they were eligible. When a group of schoolboys, who had not committed any recorded offence up to 1929, were checked twenty years later, it was found that 51 per cent had been arrested in the intervening period for various offences, excluding traffic violations. It seems unlikely that these men had never committed offences as juveniles. In England, too, Mays (1954) found that among eighty boys attending a dockland boys' club in Liverpool, which had quite strict standards that might have kept severely antisocial boys away, 42·5 per cent had convictions, another 27·5 per cent admitted having committed indictable offences without being found out, and a further group had committed less serious offences; 78 per cent were 'either officially delinquent or straying across the dangerous threshold of delinquency'.

Kobrin (1951) pointed out that in such areas where one-half or two-thirds of boys were officially delinquent, not to mention those who were not detected, the categories of delinquent and non-delinquent have little real meaning. Every boy must be exposed to a fairly evenly balanced set of values; occasionally or for definite periods he will cross the line. Kobrin went on to describe two different types of area. In one there were many successful adult offenders, with a system of crime so well organized that it penetrated the political structure. The honest leaders of society could not altogether dispense with the support of such shady adults, who often acquired social status by joining the councils of churches, charities, and other good causes. For the juveniles in such areas there was a way into the world of adult white-collar crime. In other areas, especially those with a large proportion of immigrants of different nationalities, where adult control was temporarily paralysed by differences in standards both of upbringing of children and of social cohesion, potentially delinquent children did not have these contacts with adult criminals or racketeers. In such areas, delinquency tends to 'acquire a wild, untrammelled character'. 'Both individually and in groups violent physical combat is engaged for its own sake, almost as a form of recreation.' The socially integrated offender of the first sort is confidently cynical about middle-class values, but these delinquents show by their violence that they react to their awareness of middle-class standards if only, as Cohen suggested, by showing a negative response.

The relevance of these observations is obvious, especially to rapidly developing countries such as some States in Africa and the Far East, where great opportunities for power and wealth are combined with much internal or external migration and an uncertainty in the dominant social system.

In their theory of 'delinquency and opportunity', Cloward and Ohlin (1959; 1961) have sought to develop and extend their views of Merton, Shaw and McKay, and Kobrin. They believe that each individual occupies a position in *both* legitimate *and* illegitimate opportunity structures. The Durkheim-Merton theory of anomie describes differences in access to legitimate goals and assumes either that access to illegitimate goals is freely available or that the question of availability is of little concern. The culture-transmission (Shaw & McKay) and differential-association (Sutherland-Cressey) theories assume that access to illegitimate means is variable, but do not recognize the significance of comparable differences in access to legitimate means. Criminal behaviour needs opportunities for learning and practice. In heavily delinquent areas, such as those described in the Chicago studies, there are great opportunities to learn such behaviour, and indeed to move into the professional criminal world. Some apparently uselessly aggressive and defiant behaviour by juveniles may be well adapted to draw attention to themselves as worthy recruits to older groups of criminals. In other areas there may be little opportunity for a delinquent solution. Cloward and Ohlin suggest that areas with a *criminal* subculture may be quite settled and integrated, with known professional criminals, fences for stolen property, and good opportunities for a frustrated boy to learn the criminal 'trade' from older generations. Other city areas with what they call a *conflict* subculture have a quite unorganized community in which transiency and instability of population are the main features. Here, there are few community opportunities for achieving either honest *or* criminal goals. It is of these areas, they suggest, that violence and gang fighting are most characteristic. Many readers could, no doubt, name the areas of their cities which are either settled but criminal, or else disorganized. Other studies (Sainsbury, 1955) have shown that suicides and some other forms of social breakdown are also concentrated in the second type of area. Cloward and Ohlin describe, as did Merton, a third form of subculture – the retreatist, linked especially with drug-addiction or alcoholism. Those who cannot succeed legitimately, but have internal prohibitions against, or no opportunity for, a delinquent solution, may give up the struggle, withdraw, and retreat to their own world of fantasy. Adolescents who take to drugs in the U.S.A., however, have often been delinquents *first* (McGee, 1962). In England, where

59

there is little drug-addiction, a large proportion of the middle-aged petty recidivists who throng the London prisons are alcoholics (Gibbens & Silberman, 1965). In these cases, one can speak of 'double failures', both in leading an honest life and in qualifying for recruitment to successful groups of criminals. So, too, in the individual adolescent delinquent one may see a 'double maladjustment', when a boy who has joined an aggressive gang finds himself required to show a degree of aggressive leadership which he cannot achieve or maintain (cf. Landis, Dinitz & Reckless, 1963).

These are some of the most widely discussed social theories of delinquency. Others, such as that of Sykes and Matza (1957), and the extensive 'norm-containment' theory of Reckless (1961a, b, c; 1962; Reckless & Shoham, 1963), will be more appropriately discussed later, as will certain social aspects of gangs. We may note, however, that they refer mainly to the origins of juvenile delinquency. They do *not* take account of the sociology of prisons and institutions for juveniles, which may have wider consequence than anything which happens in the outside world. Prison life is a specially constructed form of 'differential association'. In spite of much imprecision, the investigation of subcultures is of great importance to criminology, since it holds out the promise of some integration between sociological and psychological or psychiatric factors. We need to concentrate upon those subcultures which have an effect upon crime, and ask ourselves such questions as how they start and are transmitted, how they may be reversed or influenced, and whether the victims of crime belong to the same subculture. Subcultures can, presumably, be revealed only by the demonstration of common attitudes or, perhaps, at a deeper level, by traits of personality. If so, it should be possible to show that the individuals composing them have a differential perception of events. In the case of violent subcultures, for example, it has been shown that individuals more readily perceive violent stimuli. We are not concerned primarily with delinquency by groups of boys. A great many juvenile offences are committed in groups of two, three, or four, but subcultural attitudes are carried within a boy himself, whether he is alone or temporarily in a group.

Some of the most clearly defined criminal subcultures are to be found in history, continuing sometimes in a modified form up to the present day. There have existed throughout history, in very different countries and cultures, rigidly and elaborately organized groups for whom serious forms of crime, including violence and murder, have constituted a way of life or a substantial element of their social and cultural pattern of behaviour. Such are, for example, various criminal tribes, delinquent gangs, and organized crime.

As influencing and controlling factors in these groups, there may enter economic, political, religious, and other components, and not infrequently several of these are inextricably interwoven in the social pattern.

The Ismailian sect or community known as the 'Assassins' (Margoliouth, 1909), which originated in the eleventh century A.D. and spread to various parts of the Middle East, was both political and religious in its nature: 'One class of disciples . . . were ready at all times to assassinate those whom the head of the order marked out for death; and in accordance with the doctrine . . . they would risk their own lives readily in making such attempts. Nevertheless, these persons received a special training qualifying them for such missions; they were taught foreign languages and the ceremonies of foreign religions, and how to adopt and maintain a variety of disguises. Hence the assassins dispatched by the "Old Man of the Mountain", in order to win the confidence of their destined victims, would play a part for a series of months, or even years. The terrible certainty with which Hasan Sabah could strike from his fortress soon enabled him to extend his possessions and make terms with various rulers.'

In India, there long existed a number of criminal gangs and tribes consisting of professional thieves and brigands who passed on their skills to their children (Dubois, 1905; Chevers, 1870). Apart from the smaller, and also more primitive and localized criminal tribes, there were two widespread and dangerous organizations, the Dacoits and the Thags (Davidson, 1911; Farquhar, 1921), which were successfully eradicated only towards the mid-nineteenth century, through the efforts and wide powers of the Imperial Government.

Some fifty years ago, Farquhar (1921) noted: 'In all parts of India today there exist . . . tribes whose regular caste-occupation is some form of crime. In each case there is a belief that some divinity has imposed on the tribe the particular type of crime

61

which it has followed. . . . A percentage of the gains is regularly dedicated to the god or goddess who gave the tribe its criminal profession.'

It was, indeed, from these general principles, as well as from the religious and political conditions of mediaeval India, that the somewhat more complex beliefs and activities of Dacoits and Thags were evolved. Thus, for Dacoits, '. . . robbery with violence was not only an occupation but a religious and caste duty. Robbery was a hereditary profession, although the ranks of the Dacoits were continually augmented from the outside. . . . Their raids were carefully planned. . . . As a rule they preferred to avoid bloodshed, but on occasion they did not scruple to take life. . . . Their raids were undertaken only when the omens were favourable, and after the exercises of religion. The deities were Kali . . . and Sorruj Deota [the sun-god]' (Davidson, 1911).

The Thags were a secret organization of robber-stranglers, which is known to have existed in India as early as the twelfth century. In this instance, also: 'Thags believed their profession to be a religious duty, and all that they did was done under the sanction of religion. They were fully convinced that the goddess Kali . . . had commanded them to strangle and to rob. . . . The neophyte, whether the son of a Thag or a new accession, was initiated in an impressive religious ceremony, and took a dread oath of absolute fidelity to the brotherhood. Before starting on the season's operations each gang met in a suitable place, and took part in a solemn act of worship. As soon as possible after every successful operation another religious ceremony was carried out. . . . At the close of each period of operations a percentage of the gains was solemnly presented to the goddess in one of her temples.

'Among the rules which guided the Thags, perhaps the most noticeable was the law that they must never strangle a woman' (Farquhar, 1921).

It is interesting to note that so great is the criminal's singleness of purpose, and so remarkable his ability to pervert to his use the faculty of human inventiveness, that when effective measures taken by the government made it increasingly risky to continue the traditional practice of *thagi* by strangulation, there emerged, to deal with this unfortunate situation, a new class of so-called 'professional poisoners' (Chevers, 1870; Naidu, 1912) who 'doped' their prospective victim by means of a narcotic and stupefying drug prepared from Datura.*

It is also important to mention the effective co-operation, or *symbiotic relationship*, which was invariably established between these criminal groups, on the one hand, and the relevant Indian authorities and local (non-criminal) population, on the other. This is well illustrated by the two following quotations. Davidson (1911) stated that *dakoiti* was '. . . prevalent in nearly every Native State, and was encouraged by the rulers, who shared in the proceeds of the robberies as the price of their toleration. The Dacoits rarely committed their depredations near their native haunts, or even within the State which harboured them. As their victims were usually strangers, the Dacoits were not the objects of fear and hatred on the part of their neighbours, who were not, therefore, anxious to betray them to the authorities.'

Similarly, Farquhar (1921), with reference to *thagi*, observed that: 'If, therefore, some of the subjects of one of these small [Native] States pursued a certain type of crime outside the limit of the State and brought back large gains, whereof they gave considerable percentages to the Government, on the one hand, and to the temples on the other, both Government and people were usually only too willing to acquiesce in the arrangement, and to do all that was possible to protect the men who brought them so much prosperity.

'These and similar facts account for the almost universal immunity which the Thags enjoyed. They were found all over India, were closely bound to one another by oath and interest, and were usually only too well able to take prompt vengeance on any who molested the brotherhood.'

It is relevant to the study of socio-cultural evolution, here to refer briefly to an interesting *recent* report (Saran, 1962) from India

---

* Sleeman (1836), who was very largely responsible for investigating, and terminating, these age-old activities, has accurately and poetically summarized the Thag's attitude: 'A Thag considers the persons murdered precisely in the light of victims offered up to the Goddess. . . . He meditates his murders without any misgivings, he perpetrates them without any emotions of pity, and he remembers them without any feelings of remorse. They trouble not his dreams, nor does their recollection ever cause him inquietude in darkness, in solitude, or in the hour of death.' And Farquhar (1921) comments, 'Never did the strength of religious faith or the extraordinary domination which religion exercises over man's moral nature find clearer illustration.'

of a gang of professional murderers for profit. Unlike most of the earlier, traditional Indian patterns that have been described above, this gang consists mainly of people of the *same tribe* (Munda and Oraon), who *kill their own tribesmen*. In the author's opinion, this phenomenon is attributable to acculturation. Great respect is shown to the leader, and, should the latter eventually become socially reintegrated, all the members of the gang will accordingly become 'respectable citizens'. It is also noteworthy that members are *not* bound together by class, caste, language, or religion (but presumably by other specific factors determining the subculture).

According to Hurston (1939) – writing only twenty-five years ago – there is (or was) a powerful secret society in Haiti, known as the 'Sect Rouge' (and by several other names), whose activities are based on certain aspects of Voodoo religion (largely derived from West Africa). This society, meeting at night, invokes the assistance of the Voodoo deities, Maître Carrefour (Lord of the Cross-roads) and Baron Cimeterre (or Baron Samedi – Lord of the Dead): after which the members go 'running and dancing along the routes hunting for victims'. When a victim – a lonely traveller – is located, he is captured and, after certain rituals, is strangled with a cord 'made from the dried and well-cured intestines of human beings who have been the victims of other raids. . . . The gut of one victim drags his successor to his death.' This is followed by a cannibalistic meal. This is yet another example of a criminal group, whose activities are entirely determined, in this case, by its selective interpretation of the native religion.

A certain number of secret societies which were essentially political in origin (e.g. as a means of resistance to political and social oppression) came into being in Europe, particularly in Southern Italy, in the nineteenth century. Of these, the most important were the Camorra of Naples and the Mafia of Sicily (Heckethorn, 1897). These latter derived increasing strength and impetus from specific political and economic conditions which proved favourable to their survival and expansion. They made full and effective use of the criminal underworld and the ex-prison population, and did not hesitate, whenever it served their interest, to resort to blackmail, extortion, violence and murder. It is hardly surprising, therefore, that they eventually developed into extremely powerful and influential criminal organizations.

In an excellent recent work on the Mafia, Lewis (1964) states: 'The Mafia stands outside Christian morality, but the uncorrupted form of the Mafia found in feudal Sicily has an iron morality of its own. No *mafioso* sees himself as a criminal, and the Mafia has always been the enemy of petty crime – and, therefore, to a limited extent, the ally of the police, both in Sicily and the United States. The organization demands blind obedience from its members, but will defend them in return through thick and thin – and in an alien land even extends its powerful protection to all immigrants of Sicilian birth.'

In this connection, Lewis also emphasizes the general acceptance, and at least, what might be called the passive support, of the Mafia on the part of the Sicilian population – another example of the type of symbiotic relationship to which reference has already been made: 'Such *mafiosi* of the old school were only criminals in the eyes of the law and of abstract justice – and in a more confused and unfocused way in those of the peasantry they exploited. To the rest of the community they were "men of respect" and of sincere if inscrutable purpose.'

This attitude, it should be noted, persists in spite of the fact that 'Far from protecting the underdog, the Mafia today has taken the place of the oppressors of old, but it still benefits from a moral climate formed in past centuries. . . . "Manliness", once a barricade raised against injustice, now serves to keep justice out.'

The remarkable transference of this organization to the United States at the turn of the century, its infiltration and subsequent influence on the American way of life, notably in local politics, and its ever-increasing role in organized crime and racketeering of all kinds in that country, can only be mentioned here, but have been fully described by Allen (1962).

Finally, it may be appropriate to mention another cultural and traditional aspect of violence and murder – the *blood-feuds* or vendettas which have existed universally and throughout history (Gray *et al.*, 1909). These feuds have frequently involved a considerable proportion of a given community, and been carried on through several successive generations.

Thus, some fifty years ago, 'In all parts of Albania the vendetta . . . is an established usage; the duty of revenge is a sacred tradition handed down to successive generations in the family, the village

65

and the tribe. A single case of homicide often leads to a series of similar crimes or to protracted warfare between neighbouring families and communities; the murderer, as a rule, takes refuge in the mountains from the avenger of blood, or remains for years shut up in his house. It is estimated that in consequence of these feuds scarcely 75 per cent of the population in certain mountainous districts die a natural death' (Bourchier, 1910).

It is interesting to note that, according to a recent report (Bujan, 1961), post-war changes in social structure in Yugoslavia have led to the disappearance of many causes of conflict which formerly might have led to crime and vendetta in an uneducated people (in Macedonia). It is said that, although such conflicts still exist, they have become very rare. The author concludes that increased 'prosperity' has altered the form of the vendetta, the motives leading to it, and its manifestations in a particularly community.

On the other hand, Clifford (1954) stated: 'Throughout the years, crimes of honour and those connected with family vendettas have been a feature of Cyprus life. There is some improvement today, but up to recent times there have been so-called "criminal" villages not only steeped in personal feuds and the concomitant violence, but also places where assassins could be hired. These murders were almost always connected with family disputes and dishonour by seduction. In such villages the inhabitants do not go out alone at night and they take elaborate precautions against attack through open doors or windows. The linking of these villages with towns and the gradual emergence of better education and more socializing influences, have done much to reduce this problem to manageable proportions.' (See also Clifford in Grygier et al., 1965, p. 210.)

In the United States, in the late nineteenth century, there was also a notorious blood-feud which lasted some fifteen years between the Hatfields and the McCoys on the Kentucky–West Virginia border; it is not precisely known how many people were killed in the process, but their number must have been quite considerable (Jones, V. C., 1948).

One of the special features of these criminal subcultures is that the larger society, unable to disperse them, develops certain methods of coming to terms with them or 'sealing them off'. Sometimes these procedures are quite traditional. The gipsies, and the tinkers in Ireland, have a reputation (whether deserved or not) for being great thieves. In Ireland it is unlucky to refuse any food or simple request to a tinker; in England one 'crosses the palm' of a gipsy with silver if one wants good luck. In modern times, the Mafia, and the secret societies which still have widespread connections in the Far East, manage to persuade the larger culture to leave them alone. Rightly or wrongly, many citizens of the United States believe in a powerful underworld which it pays the ordinary citizen to leave in peace. In North Africa today there are 'bandit markets' in many towns. Young people, usually aged 15–20, meet after dark in quite large thieves' markets to barter stolen goods with one another, and would appear to operate with the complicity of the police. In the contemporary world, one of the main problems is to account for the conversion of accepted and traditional teenage behaviour into 'delinquent' behaviour. In North-west Africa there is an old tradition that adolescents at the time of initiation ceremonies go off into the bush, stealing a sheep for slaughter as they go; the owner never objects, for the boys will later work in his fields free of charge as a compensation. Nowadays, however, these gangs will steal and rob quite indiscriminately on these occasions. University students in Scotland, who have always had traditional 'rags' at certain times of the year, now break up graduation ceremonies with destructive horseplay and insult (verbally and physically) distinguished visitors, or their newly installed chancellor. In England, crowds returning from horse races or football matches, who have always enjoyed a great deal of tolerance of their high-spirited and intoxicated behaviour, now go to the lengths of slashing the seats of railway trains and breaking lamp-bulbs so that thousands of pounds' worth of damage is done, and it has become necessary for the railway authorities to refuse to supply the special trains for such events. The teenage riots in Germany and England, occurring in association with some stage or cinema performance, or at times quite spontaneously (Bondy *et al.*, 1957), go beyond acceptable bounds. In Japan, the adult population is mystified by the erratic and violent behaviour of teenagers, which, some years ago, was frequently influenced by their abuse of stimulant drugs of the amphetamine type. This abuse necessitated the introduction of legal control of these drugs, and, for similar reasons, a law was passed in England in 1964, with the purpose of suppressing the unauthorized possession of amphetamines.

An important aspect of this behaviour is that the parent culture not only cannot understand it, but is baffled and annoyed by it. In the past, its experimental quality was given an amused toleration; now, in its excess of violence, it arouses fear and resentment. One consequence is that nearly all teenage behaviour of an eccentric kind tends to be regarded by adults as delinquent; with the unfortunate result that such a wholesale condemnation must do much to produce and maintain the type of rebellion against established order that it aims to prevent.

What causes these changes is largely a matter of conjecture. Where the culture changes so rapidly that there are no longer recognized traditional boundaries for teenage behaviour, young people will evolve their own norms and, consequently, become confused about their role in society. These phenomena may be related to the large proportion of adolescents in the total population. Adult self-centredness and preoccupation with the enjoyment of prosperity or industrial growth may lead to a neglect of young people. Some countries, such as Israel, seem to be more successful than the Western countries in involving young people in the culture and persuading them to take part in national development.

Delinquency has a different significance in different groups, though adults tend to disregard the distinctions. Some – the so-called 'proving' offences – involve excitement and competitiveness, such as driving away cars, and some types of competitive shoplifting and souvenir hunting. Others arise from bitterness and frustration. In Nigeria, some delinquent groups are largely composed of boys who have been rejected from school because they failed to come up to educational standards. Others consist of youths who, forced to migrate on their own because of socio-economic conditions, band together in the cities.

Some of the most important consequences of rapid cultural change are to be seen in the Chinese culture of Taiwan. Here, the emergence of a youth culture is now quite new, and largely the consequence of a conflict between traditional concepts and the ever-increasing impact of Westernization. Formerly, youth received no special recognition. Children were treated very permissively until the age of six, and were then subjected to rather strong discipline until the age of fifteen, when they became semi-adults. Adults controlled their fate, arranging marriage for them, and so on. There was no period of adolescence. With the introduction of Western ideas of individual liberty and the importance of the individual, there was greater awareness of the needs of youth. But there was no acceptable way of expressing this in the culture; it could only be expressed in rebellious, violent, and antisocial ways. Reference will be made later to the evolution, in more recent times, of two distinct types of delinquent youth in Taiwan (Lin, 1958): the traditionalists, who are delinquent within the old culture, and are understood, if not accepted, by the older generation; and the modernists (often the children of the middle class), looking to the West in clothes and customs, whose behaviour is quite novel and baffling to the parent generation. A similar pattern has emerged in Japan (De Vos & Mizushima, 1959; 1962) and possibly also in several countries in South-east Asia.

This is perhaps only an exaggerated version of the trend recognizable throughout the West to differentiate a teenage culture. Formerly, there was only an 'awkward age' between puberty and adult life in which the adolescent was emphatically an aspirant adult. Today, there is a distinct phase between puberty (which occurs earlier) and adult life, long-deferred by the needs of higher education and psychological maturation processes, to which the adolescent is required to make a separate adjustment. In the West, this period has almost certainly been artificially defined and stimulated by commercial interests, which have discovered that, today, the 'teenager' from fifteen to twenty-one has a larger uncommitted spending power than the adult. Special products and special advertising seek to persuade the teenager of his or her individuality, and the social importance of fashions at this age provides a profitable if risky field for marketing.

This teenage culture has little to do with delinquency (unless the adult in his perplexity thinks of all teenagers as delinquent), but it probably alters the pattern of behaviour which delinquents adopt, and perhaps the time taken to adjust them to adult society. And it probably gives rise to certain fashions in eccentric behaviour – in drug addiction, sexual perversion or promiscuity, and crimes of excitement which are relatively new. One of the most distinct forms of contemporary subculture with a strong tendency to crime is the *subculture of violence* described by Ferracuti and Wolfgang (1963). These authors suggest that 'there is a segment both apart from, and

69

a part of, our dominant culture that places positive merit in the use of violence in interpersonal relations, that not only tolerates but even encourages or prescribes physical aggression and assaultive conduct under certain life situations. So deeply internalized are these norms and the violence value, that they have become an integral part of the personality structure of the individuals who share in and are committed to them.'

A most serious, and fortunately unique, pattern of widespread criminal violence is the so-called *violencia política* ('political violence') which, for some fifteen years, has been endemic in certain regions of Colombia (Saavedra & Rave, 1963). These activities had their (at least, more immediate) origins in political dissension, where the temporarily dominant political faction would seek completely to subdue and exterminate its defeated rivals – a pattern which was, of course, perpetuated by the opposing faction when, in its turn, it came to power. In some areas, such as Tolima, there have been recorded as many as 64 homicides per 100,000 population per year.

Ruthless as were these actions of mass intimidation and extermination, they were, therefore, at first, more essentially 'political'. Subsequently, however, there developed a number of criminal bands which on political pretexts (and exploited and encouraged, no doubt, according to well-established historical precedent, for political ends) have proceeded to carry out their 'guerilla' activities, principally in the remote rural and mountainous areas, where they can strike rapidly and then hide out in inaccessible mountain retreats. The violent crimes perpetrated by these bands of brigands invariably consist in robbery, sexual assault and murder, terrorizing and driving out the local population, and destroying or taking over their land and property.

It is significant that a large number of the recruits of these bands were children of 6–15 years of age when they themselves were compelled to witness the torture, rape, and murder of their parents, brothers, and sisters. In consequence of the indelible impression left by such early experiences, they are, not surprisingly, only too ready to seek revenge, as well as material gain. Thus they perpetuate the pattern of ruthless violence, through the seeds of violence and terror that were planted in their own childhood and adolescence.

This widespread criminal activity is strongly reinforced by very poor socio-economic conditions. The latter are, to an appreciable extent, the result of extensive arson and destruction in the agricultural areas, and the driving of threatened village populations towards the cities, where there is already much unemployment. The men will, consequently, tend to join such brigand bands also for economic reasons, and the women will try to make a living from prostitution.

Other factors than those mentioned above are, of course, also important in contributing to this picture of social disruption. Among the delinquent groups, 80 per cent are totally illiterate, as compared with 46 per cent of the general population. The great variability in social standards, common to many Latin-American countries, is very marked. The poor economic status of the majority is, therefore, inherent in the typical two-class structure of such countries: in Colombia, 70 per cent of the population live in rural areas, while 5 per cent of the population own more than half of the workable (agricultural) land. Although there are abundant natural resources (petrol, gold, platinum, etc.), they remain under the control of foreign interests. In general, capital accumulates, needless to say, 'in very few hands' (*en muy pocas manos*).

It is, however, very relevantly pointed out in the above-mentioned article, that these contributory socio-economic factors are by no means specific to Colombia and, indeed, that they constitute an even more acute problem in certain other Central and South American countries where they have, nevertheless, *not* given rise to similar endemic outbreaks of violence. Nor is it possible (as the authors rightly emphasize) to attribute this widespread criminality to social and political change, because the criminal groups in Colombia are not striving for social and political reform and progress, and the crimes they commit do not depend upon such ideals.

Chapter IV

INTERNAL AND EXTERNAL CONTROLS

The development of the sociological theories outlined briefly in the previous chapter, and the attempt to make them as all-inclusive as possible, has led to increasing consideration not only of individual, but also of the wider social and cultural, variations.

These considerations have given rise to the view that delinquency is due to a failure of either 'internal' (individual) controls or 'external' (social) controls on behaviour, or of both. We are concerned here essentially with the social and cultural influences controlling behaviour.

In considering this concept of internal and external controls, it is, however, most important to realize that there are individual *and* cultural aspects of *both* kinds of control. They do not correspond to a simple dichotomy of the psychological and the sociocultural approach. Psychiatrists, with their knowledge of the complexity of the personality, are apt to overlook the cultural aspects of personal relationships and take a very over-simplified view of the 'social environment'. Similarly, sociologists, on the one hand, tend to take an over-simplified view of mental mechanisms – e.g. Sykes and Matza's (1957) restatement in sociological terms of the psychological process of 'rationalization' of delinquent conduct can hardly be regarded as a sufficient 'theory of delinquency'. On the other hand, sociologists tend to withdraw too completely from any due consideration of those personality disorders which have a clearly established organic basis.

In fact, the behaviour and social adjustment of the epileptic boy are profoundly affected, for example, by the over-anxious and over-protective attitude of most Western parents (Pond, 1961); or, alternatively, by the attitude prevalent in certain preliterate cultures, where this condition is regarded by the parents and community as proof of magical or divine powers (Eliade, 1951).

It is, therefore, most interesting to note that not only in a country like Peru, where there is a remarkably high prevalence of convulsive disorders, and widespread illiteracy, does the general population

72

show 'frank rejection of epileptics' (Caravedo, 1959); but that, in England, where the prevalence of epilepsy is very appreciably lower, and the general standard of education very considerably higher, it is similarly recorded that 'the public have long cherished the belief that epilepsy is synonymous with mental deficiency and uncontrollable criminal impulses ... and the epileptic is thus too often treated as a pariah' (Cohen of Birkenhead, 1958).

Large-scale patterns of attitudes may be profoundly influenced, as in the Nazi youth in Germany, not so much by culture as by a small number of individuals who deliberately impose a system. (Of course, there may be dominant cultural trends, at any given time, which provide a fertile and malleable medium which is fully exploited by the oligarchy.) Thus, a German adolescent in the Hitler Youth stated: 'I took part in everything, and what I did not take part in myself, I knew of and condoned by my silence. . . . I slipped into all the things which went on in the Hitler Youth. . . . I didn't think there was anything wrong in it. . . . I merely joined in, did what everyone did' (Siemsen, 1940). Few young people could or would have failed to conform to the pattern that was both imposed and accepted. Dicks (1944–5; 1947) made a detailed report upon the psychology of German prisoners of war, Nazi and anti-Nazi. Deserters were characterized by self-centredness and resentment, and an attitude of being against all social groups: their anti-Nazi views merely happened to coincide with the views of the Allies. The anti-Nazi non-deserters, however, maintained one or more special bonds with their group – honour as a soldier, a feeling of being 'German', and other ethical scruples. 'The lack of such scruples in the deserter series stamps them as social "outsiders".'

Some of the most interesting observations upon the influence of culture on personality development have come from the anthropologist. As Alexander (1942) observed, 'the family can thus be considered a microcosm in which the cultural trends of the larger society to which the family belongs are reflected with some accuracy'. Gregory Bateson's and Margaret Mead's (1942) brilliant studies of Balinese families, and the reports of Allison Davis and John Dollard (1940) on the personality development of the Negro youth in the urban South, threw a new light upon the influence of culturally determined parental attitudes on the formation of personality. As Margaret Mead (1935) observes in her important comparative study

73

of three primitive societies in New Guinea: 'Each simple homogeneous culture can give scope to only a few of the varied human endowments, disallowing or penalizing others too antithetical or too unrelated to its major emphases to find room within its walls . . . each new generation is shaped, firmly and definitely, to the dominant trends.' She described the relationship between culturally determined attitudes and practices affecting social institutions, family structure, relations between the sexes, and the rearing of children, and its importance in influencing the development of the specific temperament and personality that characterizes the large majority of the members of a given society. The Arapesh is 'a co-operative society . . . those who find the social scheme the least congenial and intelligible are the violent, aggressive men and . . . women. . . . With their lack of distinction between male and female temperament, the same temperament suffers in each sex.' Mundugumor society, on the other hand, is not organized into a genuine co-operative community; but 'social organization is based upon a theory of a natural hostility that exists between all members of the same sex . . . the Mundugumor man-child is born into a hostile world . . . in which most of the members of his own sex will be his enemies, in which his major equipment for success must be a capacity for violence, for seeing and avenging insult, for holding his own safety very lightly and the lives of others even more lightly'. '. . . The easy-going, responsive, warm parental woman, like the easy-going, responsive, warmly parental man, is at a social discount. On the other hand, there are other aberrant personalities who are so violent that even Mundugumor standards have no place for them.'

Lowes Dickinson (1945) said of Spartan youth: 'The infants were encouraged from the beginning in the free use of their limbs, unhampered by swaddling-clothes, and were accustomed to endure without fear darkness and solitude, and to cure themselves of peevishness and crying. At the age of seven, the boys were taken away from the charge of their parents and put under the superintendence of a public official. Their education, on the intellectual side, was slight enough . . .; but on the moral side it was stringent and severe. . . . To accustom them early to the hardships of a campaign, they were taught to steal their food from the mess tables of their elders; if they were detected, they were beaten for their clumsiness and went without their dinner.'

It is in the comparative study of child-rearing practices in different societies and subgroups, which have been greatly extended in recent years (Soddy, 1955–6; Tanner & Inhelder, 1956–60), that we must look for the origins of the internal controls on behaviour which become incorporated in the individual personality. Riesman (1950), referred to above, described three types of culture, the 'tradition-directed', exemplified by primitive societies, the 'inner-directed', in which children are given general principles of conduct applicable to changing and unforeseen circumstances, and the 'other-directed' in which there is a growing tendency to model oneself on those around one, not to appear different. These he related to the length of life-expectancy and to material security which might accelerate or delay the arrival of adult status. Others have referred to 'guilt-cultures', in which guilt is induced for any deviant behaviour, and 'shame-cultures', in which disapproval from those in the socio-cultural environment is the main sanction (cf. Grinder & McMichael, 1963).

It is not possible here to describe in detail the many studies, based either on human or animal experiment, or on psycho-analytic investigation, of the process of internalization of norms and development of conscience, by which the individual child develops inner controls upon his behaviour. Indeed, there is not as yet any coherent and generally accepted theory, but rather a series of disjointed observations from many different points of view. The process is almost certainly very complicated, even if the end-product seems to come about smoothly. Though parental attitudes are frequently reflected in their children, there are so many exceptions—the atheist alcoholic father producing the religiously devout teetotaller, the preacher producing the sexually promiscuous dilettante – that the process must have many vicissitudes, even without involving the problem of genetic differences. Nevertheless, it will not be denied that a variety of factors – organic and biological, inherited or acquired – often produce a confusingly mixed aetiology in the individual case; these biological factors also vary with growth and age. Controls on conduct can clearly be internalized in the most irregular way – the armed robber, who believes that anyone who resists him deserves to get shot, may pale with horror at the thought of seducing a girl or even of practising masturbation. Some controls are internalized so completely as to withdraw certain conduct from the will of the individual; others are lightly held and easily 'eroded' unless strongly supported from outside. Psychiatrists insist that the lack of control manifested in delinquency is often closely connected with an *over*-massive internalization of controls in other areas of the personality. The fact that this great inequality of inner controls is so often to be seen in seriously deviant individuals, dating from a time when they had no opportunity of being influenced by anyone but those in the immediate circle, suggests that considerable variations occur in normal people.

It seems certain that consistency and persistence are needed if controls are to be adequately internalized. Situations, and the appropriate method of dealing with them, must recur regularly enough to enable the child to develop concepts of conduct and differentiate suitable and unsuitable responses. McCord and McCord (1959), in their important study of parental influences on a series of children before these developed in a normal or delinquent direction, showed that firm, love-oriented discipline, and also consistent but harsh discipline, produced a less than average quota of delinquents, even if the latter type may have had other undesirable effects. Passive and ineffectual fathers, who might be expected to provide an inadequate model for the growing boy, and who have frequently been blamed in recent years for delinquency in their children, also did not produce many delinquents, provided the mother was efficient. Passive and ineffectual mothers, however, frequently had delinquent children, indicating perhaps that the major part of early consistent teaching falls upon the mother and also that the young child cannot easily distinguish between an ineffective mother and one who is actively negligent and lacking in affection. The parents' behaviour towards the child, and the role model they present to the child, which may or may not be compatible, also play a variable part. Criminal fathers do not necessarily produce delinquent children.

That both parents, separately and in their relation to one another, have to be considered is a further complication. Talcott Parsons (1947) has suggested that, where controls have been very largely inculcated by the mother, the boy may associate 'good behaviour' with femininity, so that after puberty he asserts his masculinity by means of 'bad' behaviour – a common motive of the so-called 'proving' offences, of which joy-riding in cars is a frequent example.

Erratic or inconsistent behaviour by parents is one of the causes

76

of extremely patchy internalization of controls. Anxiety about the varied consequences of behaviour, or fear that things may go wrong for no detectable reason, as well as feelings of anger and hostility toward the parent that it is too dangerous to express, may give rise to the impulsiveness and inability to postpone the immediate satisfaction of desires that are so characteristic of the delinquent. Life has taught him that if a chance of present satisfaction is postponed, it may not recur; promises of rewards in the future are not fulfilled. Delinquents have also been thought to show a disturbed sense of time, an inadequate understanding of the future consequence of behaviour, as well as a poor appreciation of the past. Great insecurity, and an inability to feel safe in the present, may restrict the delinquent's attention to a constant watchfulness on the present. In order to relieve anxiety, he commonly takes refuge in a facile and frivolous cheerfulness, with a philosophy that everything is a matter of good luck or bad luck, that there are no regularities or reliable expectations.

The quality of internal controls also depends upon consistency in emotional attitudes, by which the child builds up an understanding of the moods, feelings, and motives of others. The conscience of the delinquent is often strong but highly personalized, consisting largely of the internalized avenging or rewarding figures of his parents. To this he may respond sharply, and in similar personal relationships; but the norms are not elaborated as principles of conduct to govern behaviour in impersonal situations. Whatever is not punished cannot, he thinks, be wrong.

In the most severely disturbed families, where inconsistency is accompanied by hostility or rejection, repeated and severe frustrations may lead, according to learning theory derived from animal experiments (Maier, 1949; Marquart, 1948; Patrick, 1934), to a breakdown of the learning process. Like the hungry rat which, presented with a problem in obtaining food that is quite insoluble, falls back ultimately upon stereotyped repetitive behaviour that does not aim at a solution, so the severely 'maladapted' delinquent (in Jenkins' (1949) phrase) and the later recidivist may commit stereotyped and repetitive crimes which have no hope of success and are not perceptibly designed to solve any of their personal problems (Scott, 1960b; Jenkins, 1949). In such cases, there may be a serious breakdown of internalized controls.

77

The basis for the development of inner controls, and the meaning of the most tenaciously held controls, may be laid down in the first five years or so, during which the child is virtually confined to the family circle. It involves consistency in action and emotional attitude, and the process of identification with parental models. The latter may vary between the 'experience model' and the 'role model' – the parents as he finds them, and as he learns to understand them in time. Many a child must learn to accommodate himself to the realization that an affectionate mother may also be promiscuous, and that an affectionate father's absences may be due to imprisonment for burglary. This is especially the case when the parents have learnt to accept one another's idiosyncrasies and intuitively transmit this understanding to the child.

After the age of five, the inner controls need to be reinforced and exercised by consistent experience, though it is not uncommon to find adult offenders who appear to have few scruples but have an ineradicable sense of guilt for their behaviour as the result of an early upbringing in the strict and rigid ethics of some religious organization, or cultural family situation. But if such internalization can occur in adult life as a result of hypnosis or the so-called 'brainwashing' techniques, it can presumably be produced during the later years of childhood. When the child begins to move outside the home, however, there are many additional factors which may reinforce or undermine controls. One has to consider not consistency in a parent, and between parents, but whether this image is consistent with what the child begins to learn about other parents. Some parents may become inconsistent when they are made aware of the attitudes of other parents in the neighbourhood, or may change their standards to achieve some consistency with surrounding society. The age at which it is considered suitable for a girl to start wearing lipstick or high heels, for example, is apt to be decided by the district or the school, or as a result of some compromise between what may be regarded as appropriate by some parents, or by the predominant local culture, respectively. Pakistani girls, who are very strictly controlled in their own culture, frequently come into conflict with their fathers in England when they get friendly with boys at fourteen or fifteen, like the English girls at school. This may bring them before a court as 'beyond control'.

A similar process frequently gives rise to the misinterpretation of the case histories of delinquents. Recidivists especially may describe their parents in most favourable terms, though older records, when they can be obtained, show that the parents' were, in fact, aggressive, rejecting, and inconsistent. At first, the child must accept his parents; later, he begins to realize that they may differ from others, and one of his motives for associating with other delinquents may be a sense of relief at finding that other boys have equally unsatisfactory parents. In late adolescence, however, with increasing independence, he grows ashamed of the defects of his parents. As his knowledge of the wider world grows, he tends to 'normalize' the parental image, describes them favourably to any observer in adult life, and may even begin to believe in this idealized concept. When the parents are dead, this idealization not infrequently amounts to 'deification' – irrespective of their nature or adequacy during their lifetime.

The culture of the school – the children's and the teacher's – is one of the first outside contacts which the child must make. The behaviour required may be new to the child, and he soon learns to perceive the status of his own parents in relation to those of other children. In recent years, attention has been paid to the cultural attitude of the teachers. Not infrequently, they themselves come from lower socio-economic classes, but have risen to a higher status by gaining scholarships, etc. They are thus particularly likely to reject certain lower-class values and to be impatient with those who do not share their social and intellectual ambitions. In some parts of Africa, such as Nigeria, the Cameroons, and Madagascar, children are liable to be confused by a type of education which emphasizes a completely alien culture; more care is needed in working out a method of re-interpreting their own culture. Unsuitable education may be accompanied by great material prosperity, but, nevertheless, give rise to a higher incidence of delinquency, especially since there is little provision for those in need of special education.

Some societies seem also to maintain their customary controls better than others in the face of various vicissitudes, such as emigration. This may depend upon patterns of family organization or cultural patterns of external control determined by religious belief and other factors. In the African village, for example, the child may be severely punished by its parents; but in the 'extended family' system there are aunts and uncles and grandparents who will intercede and offer alternative identifications for the child. In exceptional cases the neighbours will intercede with the parents. This is a pattern very easily lost in conditions of urbanization and industrialization, where economic conditions may lead to the two-parent or even one-parent family – the small 'nuclear' family of Western countries.

Even though the internal controls may be established in the same way in most cultures, some of these may offer the expectation that they will be supported and extended by external controls and others may not. In China, for example, it has been said that Confucianism offered a secure role for everyone; each had his place in society and could feel secure in it. The Chinese child could expect that inner control would be supported by external control on behaviour. Much will depend, however, upon whether the culture has a flexible or rigid framework of expectations. In many cultures the child can expect that inner controls will be regularly reinforced by orderly external controls, by traditional patterns of behaviour. In others, such as the United States, however, the emphasis is upon individuality and self-responsibility. The child is taught, implicitly or explicitly, that he must stand upon his own feet, make his own future. The marshal's baton is in every haversack; anyone can be President. Societies which provide few formal external controls upon behaviour must rely mainly upon the strength of early inner controls. It may be a feature of all industrialized and urbanized communities to overstrain these inner controls.

One of the characteristics of the 'good' boy, even in a delinquent area, as Reckless has pointed out, is that he has a good 'self-concept' (Reckless, Dinitz & Murray, 1956). Certain sorts of behaviour are ruled out as being not characteristic. He 'would not do such a thing'. He may even think that he 'would not dream of doing this' (though psycho-analysts would say that this is exactly what he might *dream* of). Thus for the growing youth, as indeed for all of us, our idea of ourselves only has meaning in a cultural context.

This function of playing a role (and indeed a variety of roles – as affectionate son, obedient pupil, responsible troop leader, and so on) makes a vital contribution to enmeshing the individual in a series of external relationships which control his behaviour. These involve him in a number of reference groups which have importance for him and give him a measure of his identity. In the middle class, where the school-fellows and friends with whom he comes in contact are (whether intentionally or not) selected to reinforce parental attitudes, these various roles are limited in number and within the capacity of the growing boy. In a complex Western society, especially in areas of a city where the parents cannot hope to exercise much supervision, the boy has to orientate himself to a great multiplicity of groups, and experiences a confusion of roles. Many men of distinction from a humble origin can remember this painful confusion of roles, when they had to be the tough fighter in the street-corner society as well as the promising scholar at the high school, with quite different roles and expectations. This conflict of roles – especially if there is some disappointment in one of them – can cause difficulties of which parents may not be aware. A peer culture which can combine these roles and resolve conflicts has great attractions, and it is not surprising that many teenagers should show a passionate attachment to a society of their contemporaries which can succeed in fulfilling this function, thus providing them with some sense of security and identity.

Spontaneous groups of adolescents clearly play a very important part either in supporting or 'eroding' norms of behaviour already established and in establishing the adolescent's attitudes to himself and his contemporaries. There are important social class differences in the formation of such groups. In the middle-class family, or the working-class family with middle-class aspirations, children are closely supervised, their friends and social contacts quietly selected for them; dependence is prolonged by further education and free time often taken up with homework. It is easy to overestimate the sociability of adolescents. In England, Logan and Goldberg (1953) studied a true sample of eighteen-year-olds called up for military service, and found that about one-quarter (excluding students) rarely went out without their parents and had a very limited social life. The Netherlands, too, has a home-bound culture, with a tendency even among adults to visit one another's homes rather than meet in public. Street-corner groups may represent a bare majority and will always include those whose homes are uncomfortable for emotional or material reasons.

The working-class boy, however, is usually driven or lured away by overcrowding, large families, and close proximity to neighbours to play in the street and take care of his younger siblings. From the age of six or seven he orientates himself to an outside world largely dictated by housing conditions; and, with many different ages represented, the older dominating the younger ones by force, the groups may be for protection as well as for play. He grows up with the 'distinctive pattern of concerns' described in America by Miller (1958) and in similar terms in England by Spinley (1953) as expecting trouble, being tough especially in enduring aggression, being smart or quick-witted in practical matters, on the look-out for excitement, believing in luck or fate, and maintaining a great show of rugged independence in spite of close emotional bonds to home. The middle-class child is protected from aggression when young and so is still scared of it in adolescence, but is trained to be stoical about separation from home (Spinley, 1953). Miller (1958) connected the working-class boy's need for autonomy to an upbringing in a female-centred home. For all adolescents at some time 'when the home carapace is shed, the group offers a shelter in which a new skin may harden – a breathing-space for the acquisition of confidence' (Scott, 1956).

The influence of gangs on delinquency is clearly a very complex problem on which purely sociological explanations may not be capable of throwing much light, since groups tend to be small and very variable in composition and interrelationship of members. Thrasher (1927), however, tended to emphasize the aspect of youthful high spirits in an atmosphere of poor family control and social disorder: as Miller (1958) puts it, 'fun, profit, glory and freedom is a combination hard to bear'. Cohen (1955), as we have seen, emphasized the opposite, the pointless, negativistic, destructive behaviour of boys who drew strength from a group which denied middle-class values and gave them a status they had lost.

How important status may be in groups of all ages is suggested by observations in Denmark (Christiansen, 1955) of those who were imprisoned for collaborating with the enemy in the Second World War. Of those collaborators who had had no previous convictions for conventional crimes, many were later reconvicted: but those who *had* had previous convictions were frequently not reconvicted. Being a political prisoner may have raised their status in the prison and their self-concept of being a member of a superior class.

Some psychologists take the view that the delinquent's gang is often only a group in default of opportunity to join more conventional groups. When studied in institutions, many boys of this kind feel extremely inadequate in all social skills, unable to communicate effectively with their contemporaries except by catch-phrases or horse-play. They may be social isolates who, rather than have no group at all, follow one another, or are manipulated by a strong personality.

It is a curious fact, which certainly calls for cross-cultural comparisons, that specifically delinquent gangs with a fairly large membership and a structure of leaders and lieutenants, etc. do not seem to exist outside the United States. London delinquents will mention with pride being associated distantly with an awe-inspiring gang, but when a research project in gang-participant social work was set up some years ago it had to be abandoned because no gang could be found. Gangs are always present in the next district, or they existed last year; never here and now. This 'mirage' effect may be an important characteristic. Yablonsky (1959) studied thirty delinquent gangs in New York, but admits that leaders' opinions about size or affiliations varied with their emotional state. In one case, 'in an hour's interview, the size of his gang varied from 100 members to 4,000, from five brother gangs or alliances to sixty'. Apart from size, however, Yablonsky's description in detailed socio-psychological terms of the inner composition and fluctuating relationships appears similar to European experiences as described by Scott (1956). The core of the gang is commonly a severely disturbed youth who needs the gang in order to deal with his personal problems of inadequacy, and works to keep it together. A second level of membership only uses the gang according to emotional needs at given times, and a third or outer ring only acknowledges any connection with it on odd occasions or 'for old time's sake'. Bordua (1961) has suggested, however, that unemployment in this age group may leave large groups available, and one might suppose that if, in heavily-industrialized countries, large cities grow up round one or two industries, a fluctuation in the industry might affect a whole age group. In Taiwan (Lin, 1958) and Japan (De Vos & Mizushima, 1959; 1962), there tends to be a differentiation between modernist or Western-oriented groups and 'traditional' gangs of lower social status.

The social psychology of the common small groups of delinquents of fluctuating type seems to represent a vital meeting-point of the social, cultural, psychological, and psychiatric aspects of delinquency. Many different relationships are seen. A group of more than three boys often includes one very dull one, grateful to find the friendship of such 'smart' and important comrades. As Scott (1956) points out, an older brother may involve in delinquency a younger brother of whom he is jealous, so as to devalue him in the parents' eyes. Yet, apart from the frequent cases where a participant delinquent gets involved quite unwittingly in a group offence, the existence of a group is a great solvent of the individual consciences of its members. Commonly, members leap-frog one another in leadership, one breaking into the house or shop, another doing the stealing, a third suggesting how to dispose of the goods, though each would fail in nerve were he required to execute the whole crime alone. Fritz Redl (1945) has suggested that the conscience-releasing factor is not so much loyalty, friendship, and solidarity (which are often not much in evidence) but the powerful stimulus of wishing one could commit an act without guilt and then seeing someone do it who clearly does not feel guilty afterwards.

Gibbens (1963) has suggested that the group, especially of older adolescents of 17–21, should be examined in relation to what it is *not*, as well as what it is. Four delinquent boys are often the residue of twenty friends at school, but the other sixteen have gradually retired from the group into individual relationships with girls and going to dances and parties. Though sexually interested and possibly active in transient relations, the gang member is forced by his inability to form affectionate socio-sexual relations, or by his experience of rejection and frustration in any such attempts, into association with others like himself. Security against sexual fears and, in delinquents, against sexual maladjustment is one function of the gang. This accounts for the important, and by no means infrequent, occurrence in juvenile gangs of latent or overt homosexual activities and group rape (Blanchard, 1959; Colin & Bourjade, 1961; De Vos & Mizushima, 1960; Franchini & Introna, 1961; Heuyer, 1954; Michaux *et al.*, 1957; Parrot & Gueneau, 1960).

The group may also help to 'erode' controls by providing ready-made methods of rationalization of motives. Sykes and Matza (1957) have recast the psychological theory of rationalization into sociological terms as group 'techniques of neutralization', of external and internal controls, which enable the boy to overcome his scruples

84

about being delinquent. Five forms of justification are commonly used: the denial of responsibility ('I didn't mean to do it'); denial of injury ('I didn't really hurt anybody'), condemnation of the condemners ('They had it coming to them'); paranoid projection of hostility ('Everyone is picking on me'); or loyalty to the group ('I didn't do it for myself'). The authors do not mention a sixth technique which many observers would regard as common, namely, the technique of 'normalization' ('Everyone does it really, and I'm no different. I'm no saint').

The work of Reckless (1961a, b, c; 1962; Reckless & Shoham, 1963) is especially pertinent to the present discussion, since in his 'norm-containment theory' he has addressed himself specifically to the question of internal and external controls. 'It has a double aspect; the capability of groups to transmit norms effectively and hold their members within bounds and the retention of norms by the individual as an inner control over behaviour. The retention aspect of norm containment can also be viewed in terms of norm erosion – the sloughing off of the moral significance of norms, the neutralization of the oughtness, the emancipation from internalized norms, etc.' (Reckless & Shoham, 1963). Starting from a consideration of the 'good' boy in a high delinquency area (Reckless, 1958; Reckless, Dinitz & Murray, 1956; 1957; 1962; Scarpitti et al., 1960), he considers that the various subcultural theories do not throw light on which boys are unaffected by these influences and which become delinquent. One may consider the norm-transmitting function of the family or group and the norm-holding capability of the group of which a boy is a member, and their various relationships. The capacity of this group to transmit the norm and to hold the individual within the bounds of expectations is decreased, he considers, by urbanization, migration, dislocation, culture conflict, political disturbance, etc. The norm-holding powers of a group might be fruitfully linked also with the observable degree of anomie, on the assumption that the containing capability of society is directly proportional to its integration of norms, its cohesion, and its solidarity.

Norm-erosion is closely connected with age. In adolescence one expects boys to cast off part of the moral content of norms which were internalized as children, and perhaps to go through a phase of sanction-oriented compliance (compliance through fear of consequences). If children before adolescence show only this sanction-oriented compliance, it is doubtful whether they will pass through the rebellion of adolescence without delinquency; but the adolescent who has only this type of compliance with norms may still draw a supple mental inner containment from such things as a strong goal-orientation, a favourable self-image, and a high frustration tolerance.

Reckless applies this theory only to 'the large middle range of juvenile and adult offenders' who break the law over a period of time; he excludes compulsive delinquents, those with severe character disorders, those who commit cultural crime, such as members of the criminal tribes of India, or those educated in a criminal career. Accidental crimes and spontaneously contagious criminal behaviour are also excluded.

'Containment theory not only describes non-causal buffers against deviation, but it also describes probability. . . . Obviously, individuals who can be classified as strong–strong (strong in external and strong in internal containment), will have a very low probability of committing crime or delinquency (becoming a legal deviant); whereas individuals who are classified as weak–weak . . . will have a very high probability of committing crime and delinquency.

'The writer is quite prepared to admit that, of the two containing buffers against deviation, the inner containment is the more important in the mobile, industrialized settings of modern society. This is because individuals in such societies spend much of their time away from the family and other supportive groups which can contain them. As a result, they must rely more on their own inner strength to function competently. It is also probable that the outer is operationally more important than the inner containing buffer, in less mobile, less industrialized societies where the clan, the caste, the tribe, the village retain their effectiveness, or in the modern, intensively managed, communistic societies. In such societies, the strength of the self, away from a circumscribed social structure, is not put to a test, and we really do not know how strong it is or how well it can manage alone' (Reckless, 1962).*

* There is a vast literature on delinquent group formation and gangs, but special reference may be made to the works of Bloch & Niederhoffer, 1958; Eynon & Reckless, 1961; Miller, 1959; Short & Strodtbeck, 1964; Whyte, 1943; Yablonsky, 1962.

Chapter V

COMPARABILITY OF STATISTICS

The hope of being able to compare the criminal statistics of one country with another has been maintained ever since the first statistics appeared in France in the mid-nineteenth century. World opinion seems to be divided between those who are frankly pessimistic and those who maintain at best a cautious optimism. Almost every page of the foregoing chapters bears witness to the difficulties of any strict comparison. The legal definitions differ, legal procedure is different, police organization and efficiency vary; above all, the level of tolerance of crime in different societies, which determines whether cases are reported to the police, is never the same.

Since 1929, the United States has had considerable experience, with the Uniform Crime Reports, in trying to achieve some uniformity in the divergent practices of the different States. Reporting cases to the police, in spite of the variations to which it is liable, is perhaps the best index of crime, recorded as 'crimes known to the police'. In 1950, the United Nations resolved to collect international data on such universally recognized offences as homicide, robbery, aggravated assault, etc.; but they met with little success in obtaining comparable statistics.

In juvenile delinquency, the tendency was first to use juvenile court statistics. But so many different courses of action are open to the police that the police statistics are today agreed to be the best. Legal classifications are particularly inappropriate for describing juvenile activity. Robbery may refer to a serious crime by a teenager, or to the activity of a small boy who takes sweets from another boy under threats from a catapult; the recorded offences make no distinction. Multiple offences, especially, are recorded differently. If three or four types of offence have been committed, then only the most serious is usually recorded; the latter may be acknowledged as the gravest threat to society, but the other offences may conceal widespread damage of another kind. If four boys commit the same offence – as is very likely if they are under the age of twelve or thirteen – this may be recorded as four offences.

Some modification of these doubts and difficulties is provided by the interesting, if baffling, international statistics of crime provided by the International Criminal Police Organization (Interpol) in Paris. Since 1950, the seventy or so countries and territories that are members of the organization have supplied statistics of crime of limited scope, but of a type which is designed to afford some broad comparability. They comprise statistics for eight groups of offences: . (1) Homicide. (2) Sex offences, grand larceny, and petty larceny. (3) Major larceny. (4) Minor larceny. (5) Fraud. (6) Counterfeiting, (7) Offences connected with drugs. (8) Total offences. In each group, in the first place, the total number of offences (including attempts) known to the police is given, together with the rate per 100,000 of the total population and the number of 'cases solved'; and, second, the number of persons 'identified' as responsible (arrested or known, but not necessarily convicted) per 100,000 total population. Reporting is variable. In 1961–2, twenty-two states contributed data to Interpol that had not done so in 1959–60, and seven countries lapsed, although they had reported in 1959–60 (namely, Colombia, Spain, Indonesia, Jamaica, Lebanon, Senegal, and Uruguay). (Interpol, 1964.)

The results are extremely interesting, though the figures themselves, as one might expect, can be regarded only as a basis for further inquiry, but they must indicate (subject to the variations in definition) major preoccupations of the states concerned (or of their ruling class) and, through them, of the police. They are thus very relevant to the subject of the present report, if not necessarily to the amount of criminal behaviour in these countries.

The first category, 'wilful murder', includes 'any kind of act performed with the purpose of taking human life, no matter in what circumstances. This definition excludes accidental manslaughter and abortion but not infanticide.' Reference to the national statistics of the United Kingdom shows that, in its report to Interpol, this country recorded 437 cases known to the police (0·94 per 100,000 population), comprising murder (148), murder of children under one year of age (11), attempted murder (204), infanticide (27), and threats to murder (47), but excluded 114 cases of manslaughter and 404 cases of 'causing death by dangerous driving.'

The world incidence in these 'murderous assaults' shows startling variations. Colombia sent no return in 1961, and Mexico sent only details about persons dealt with (who amounted to 11,302 or 30·3 per 100,000 population). Burma headed the list with a reported rate of 39·2 per 100,000. But though 8,000 cases were reported and 4,000 'solved', 17,000 persons were 'responsible' for these attacks, or 81·4 per 100,000. This might suggest, but almost certainly does not mean, that every attack involved four people! Rather remarkably, the neighbouring state of Cambodia reported 15 cases among six million inhabitants (0·25), and Laos 60 for three millions (or 2·0 per 100,000); but Thailand reported a rate of 20·38. The next leading countries were the Philippines (17·16), Bolivia (15·8), Uganda (13·5), and Cyprus (13·0). European countries gave a very low rate of murderous assaults; all, except France, vary between 0·5 and 3·0 per 100,000. France is reported to have the exceptionally high rate of 7·31 – equal to that of Pakistan (7·25), and the United Arab Republic (7·9). Both these countries, however, have an 'arrest' rate for individuals which is more than double the rate of 'cases reported', e.g. in Pakistan 6,812 cases were reported, 4,925 cleared up; but 15,399 persons were dealt with (a rate of 16·41). The high rate reported in France is almost certainly an artefact of definition; the arrest rate of 3·75 was considerably lower than the 'cases known', and included no less than 77 juveniles, a unique feature in world statistics.

Sexual offences are given the following definition: 'Each country will base its reports on its own laws in determining whether an act is a sex crime or not, it being understood that rape and trafficking in women shall always be included.' However defined, the interesting fact that emerges is that there is an inverse relationship between reports of sex crimes and reports of murderous assault – at least in extreme cases – as the table on page 90 shows.

Sex crimes commonly cause concern to the public and the police and to legislators in the developed countries – especially, perhaps, in Protestant countries, in which the murder rate is usually exceptionally low. Countries with very high homicide rates report few sexual crimes. A possible explanation – following Durkheim's (1895) proposition – is that communities in which the sanctity of human life is generally accepted and respected will turn their attention to somewhat less threatening forms of deviation, namely, sexual offences. In some countries, such as Ghana, Nigeria, Nyasaland, Kenya, and the Solomon Islands, sex crimes are at least more

Crimes known to the Police, per 100,000 population

Country	Sex Crimes	Homicide and Attempted Homicide
Germany	110·9	2·1
Denmark	80·9	1·3
New Zealand	71·5	0·89
Australia	71·8	2·07
Netherlands	66·9	2·2
Fiji	58·0	3·0
Austria	55·0	2·0
Switzerland	53·4	0·47
Canada	44·3	2·0
United Kingdom	43·7	0·9
Sweden	43·0	0·5
Uruguay	43·0	6·6
France	29·5	7·31
Philippines	10·6	17·16
Bolivia	10·4	15·79
Thailand	10·34	20·38
Mexico	13·3	31·0
Burma	16·9	39·2

commonly reported than murderous assaults. One might postulate that this reflects the influence of external legal systems, to which these countries have all been subjected. In the U.S.A. the number of sex crimes reported is almost exactly twice that of murderous assaults. But in several countries of the Middle East and Southern Asia, United Arab Republic, Ceylon, Pakistan, India, Thailand and the Philippines (but *not* Malaya) there are fewer sex crimes reported or dealt with than homicidal assaults. Laos reported nine sex crimes among three million population.

Apart from homicidal attacks and sex crimes, a third most interesting aspect of these statistics refers to offences involving drugs. Although they may have a very doubtful significance in terms of behaviour, they certainly raise interesting questions about police practice and community attitudes. Offences reported or coming to the notice of the police must, presumably, indicate the extent to which they are publicly condemned or else condoned or concealed. In most of the countries of the Western world, the number of cases of arrests for narcotics offences is small. In Hong Kong, however, it is the commonest offence; 15,000 cases are reported and 12,000 dealt with – a rate of 444·3. In Burma (138·6), Ceylon (38·7), Thailand (34·6), and Singapore (33·0), these are among the most frequent cases to be reported and arrested. In the Philippines, however, it either is not, or is not considered to be, a serious problem – only 73 cases per year were arrested (0·26). In the United Arab Republic (Egypt) it is the most common offence (20·4) apart from minor larceny, and it is also important in the Sudan; in all these countries it must absorb a great deal of the time and energy of the police forces.

These statistics have been discussed from the point of view of the interest they arouse rather than that of their doubtful or uncertain significance. It is often said that they have little value when one country is compared with another, but that they indicate genuine trends in any one country from one year to the next with greater certainty. Opinions on this question are divided; whether trends are reliably indicated may itself vary from country to country – depending upon the stability of definition and of administrative practice. Legislative change is often preceded by a fairly prolonged period of practical or administrative modification.

Faced with this dilemma, Sellin and Wolfgang (1964) have evolved an interesting method which could be used in principle as a basis for international comparisons. Their aim was to achieve a measurement of crime. In essence, they obtained fairly detailed descriptions of some 140 types of criminal act, covering every type of crime. These were shown to large groups of police, students, and juvenile court magistrates, with the request that they attach a 'score' to each offence to indicate their assessment of its gravity. There was very substantial agreement between these groups, though the magistrates tended to take a slightly more lenient view than the police of some offences and, on the whole, the estimates of gravity come close to the attitude implied in the penal law and the penalties which it provides. A minor theft will score '1', for example; but taking the same amount of money by armed robbery counts '11', with the threat of violence counting '4' towards the score; murder counts 26 times as much as a simple theft. In this way it is possible to say

91

that public opinion attaches a certain average weight to the damaging element in any particular crime – whether injury to people, the threat of injury, the loss due to theft or damage to property, or offences against public order. One can attach a certain score to each of a series of offences and give a numerical value to the total 'damage' which they are considered to entail. Two towns may record the same number of crimes in a year, but it is possible on the basis of such scores to say that one town's aggregate of crime was two or three times more serious than that of the other. If it could be shown that two countries attached the same value to the scale of offences, then one would have a measure for comparing their respective criminality.

An investigation of opinion in European countries, such as is now being undertaken, might possibly reveal considerable agreement in the 'value' attached to crimes, but it is almost certain that some countries would show marked differences in this respect and that rapidly developing countries such as Nigeria would show shifting values in a relatively short time. In a paper on 'The African View of Crime', Clifford (1964) describes the attitudes of rural and still tribal Africans in Northern Rhodesia, as compared with the shifting values of the urban African who has been brought up in detachment from the tribal attitudes and controls, but has not yet established an adequate and stable adjustment to the new socio-cultural conditions, The author asked groups of these Africans to make a list of what they considered to be crimes. The number of 'mentions' was as follows:

Murder	17	Other sex crimes	4
Stealing	14	Burglary and breaking-in	4
Fighting and assault	14	Robbery	2
Adultery	10	Malicious damage	2
Rape	4		

To the rural African, acts which disturb the fabric of social relationships are worse than those which affect individuals; as mentioned above, criminal acts committed against individuals outside the tribal group may be entirely condoned or even encouraged. Adultery, which acutely disturbs kinship relations, is regarded very seriously. Failure to appease the ancestors might well be construed as a social wrong or a crime. The individual counts for less than the social group.

A system of measurement, such as that of Sellin & Wolfgang

(1964), would have great value not only in establishing international comparisons, but in providing information about the success or failure of corrective treatment. Using their method in England for the study of failure rates of juveniles after discharge from institutional treatment, Scott (1964) showed how it may introduce qualitative detail into the crude and relatively meaningless fact that 65 per cent were reconvicted in three years. Scoring the 210 offences of 100 'failures', he showed that 58 did not have any score at all on the basis of theft, injury, or damage, e.g. offences such as loitering: it is a defect of the Sellin-Wolfgang system that it does not measure 'intention', which has some importance for society. Classifying offences rated '2' or below as trivial, and '3' or above as serious, the following results were obtained in the 210 offences:

Classification of offences	No.	%
Trivial:		
0 and all offences scored '1'	89	43
All the '2's and below	156	74
Serious:		
All the '3's and above	54	26
All the '5's and above	16	8

Unless a ruling minority is repressing crime in any country, very common offences will usually be lightly punished by the courts. In the same country there may be wide differences according to the frequency of offences. In the centre of London's shopping area, for example, shoplifting is very common and is nearly always punished by a fine in the first instance; in outlying areas, where there is less shoplifting, it is more often punished by imprisonment or heavier fines (Gibbens & Prince, 1962). And it is implied by the theory of subcultures that those who share in a subculture of violence, for example, will attach slighter importance to aggressive offences than will the wider community.

Chapter VI

LEARNING AND UNLEARNING

The problem facing those who study delinquency is to find out how children learn to become delinquent or fail to learn to be law-abiding; and, in treating the delinquent, how he may be educated or re-educated.

It is commonly said, for example by Sykes and Matza (1957), that 'it is now largely agreed that delinquent behaviour, like most social behaviour, is learned, and that it is learned in the process of social interaction'. But there can surely be few statements about human behaviour which, expressed in such absolute terms, are acceptable. Presumably, there is a small area of human behaviour, such as some aspects of sexual behaviour, which is largely instinctive even if it occurs always in some social context. If it is meant that 'most delinquent behaviour, like other social behaviour, is learned', then the proposition would be strongly supported by those who took part in the Topeka Conference. Even instinctive behaviour cannot occur more than once without the involvement, in its repetition, of both experience and some learning process.

It was suggested, earlier in this report, that the Sutherland-Cressey theory of differential association was perhaps the most acceptable theory of the causation of crime because it did not appear to say more than that crime was learned behaviour; learned, as Sutherland said '. . . by all the mechanisms that are involved in any other learning' (Sutherland & Cressey, 1955). Such a qualification would satisfy most psychiatrists that all they believe about the psychological origins of crime is also included in causation, for, even if the mechanisms are different, an individual can be said to 'learn' to make neurotic responses at an early age, and these may play a large part in distorting the learning processes which are involved in later social interaction. No one can make an exclusive claim for one form of learning as opposed to another, and the theory has value in stressing the continuity and interpenetration of personal, social, and cultural factors.

Some psychiatrists may well feel that to use 'learning' in this wide sense is to take away the accepted meaning of the word as implying a deliberate lesson being consciously taught and learnt; indeed, that to use it in the wider sense may give a false impression of unanimity by papering over what they conceive to be a large cleft between the concepts of sociologists and psychiatrists. But if there was one result that emerged with particular clarity from the Topeka Conference, it was that, in considering delinquency as a problem of learning and unlearning, the participants found a common approach that permitted a free and constructive interchange of concepts and ideas between the several disciplines concerned.

It is implicit in this approach that there cannot be any sharp dichotomy between the personal and the cultural aspects of the individual – the 'psychiatric' and the 'social'. Just as there is a unique aspect to the social attitudes of the individual, so, too, even the most deeply internalized aspects of his personality will reflect cultural pehnomena. One may draw an analogy between this general situation and the phenomenon of *prejudice* as it occurs in the community (Allport, 1954; Unesco, 1956a; cf. also Kisker, 1951; Klineberg, 1950; Unesco, 1957). Thus, for example, in studies of attitudes of discrimination against people of a particular race, colour, or creed, four types of individual can be demonstrated. There are those who are personally prejudiced and who also openly discriminate against the minority; but there are also strongly prejudiced individuals who, because of allegiance to some wider social group or set of principles, are not willing to show discrimination. Conversely, there are some who are unprejudiced and do not discriminate, but there are also those who feel that they must discriminate out of loyalty to a discriminating group. There is a personal *and* a cultural aspect of both the inner prejudice and the outer discrimination in behaviour.

This example suggests that a distinction must be drawn between direct and indirect learning. Clearly, there are situations in society or in family life in which direct examples are taught or demonstrated. Indirect learning, however, plays an important part in the origins of delinquency. Conflict between parents who are demonstrating opposing ideas, or a parental pattern of 'Don't do as I do; do as I say', may indirectly teach lessons which are precisely the opposite of what is intended. These forms of indirect learning are universally recognised as important factors in the causation of delinquency.

Apart from insoluble conflicts in parental attitudes presented to the child, there may be similar conflicts between the reconcilable attitudes of home, and the irreconcilable attitudes of the social world outside, such as one finds in the sons of admirable and lovable but criminal fathers. The existence of direct and indirect learning suggests that unlearning may also be of two kinds.

Much depends also upon the existence of cultural patterns of learning, the extent to which there are well-recognized patterns of apprenticeship in social relations. The growing boy soon recognizes the existence of those expectations of learning, and associates them with age. The undergraduate does not expect that he will still think it appropriate to take part in an irresponsible 'rag' when he has graduated. One has found many eighteen-year-old delinquents who, when asked to describe the next five years, will say, for example, that when they have finished military service they 'will marry and settle down'. They feel that delinquency is compatible with their present age-status, but not with adult married status. Criminals' autobiographies of the past and the expected future often reveal unusual attitudes and expectations, and a cross-cultural comparison of these expectations would be interesting.

Hitherto, we have considered the cultural factors in learning delinquent patterns of behaviour in the open community, with the social forces which lead to a boy's first appearance in court. But some 60–80 per cent of delinquents appear only once in court. Though these temporary delinquents are numerically important and influence all studies of the social origins of crime, it does not follow that the causes of recidivism and serious delinquency are necessarily the same, or that they differ only quantitatively. When learning *and* unlearning are considered together, one cannot limit consideration to the wider social background of the unconvicted offender, but must also necessarily consider the penal process as a cause of both learning and unlearning of criminal behaviour.

The prison or reformatory culture as a training-ground for further crime is so wide and important a subject that it cannot be dealt with fully in a brief report of this kind. It has long been recognized (Howard, 1784), and remains equally true today, that, as a school for crime and as a criminal subculture, the reformatory or prison probably has no equal. In Taiwan, and many other parts of the world, delinquents refer to penal institutions as 'college'. Some would say that the penal process, however necessary it may be for the maintenance of some external controls for the non-offender, inevitably places the offender under an additional handicap. The majority of those who go to an institution for the first time have the strength to avoid further crime in spite of this added handicap; for those who have not this strength of personality (internal controls), it merely loads the dice more heavily against their subsequent chances of an adequate social adjustment. If the offender responds favourably, it may be in spite of, rather than because of, penal methods and corrective treatment as they are commonly applied.

The element of truth in such views is so obvious that there is perhaps some risk that they may lead to excessive despair or cynicism. There is in institutions a conflict of forces tending to contribute towards either the learning or else the unlearning of delinquency; but most delinquents are not reconvicted after the age of twenty-five (even if in spite of, rather than because of, penal procedures); it might, therefore, be sufficient to hold these forces in even balance – merely to 'do no harm', to enable constructive or maturational changes to occur (as with the 'masterly inactivity' advocated by the older physicians).

At least it can be said that the 'unlearning' processes are the ones which can be studied. It may be very difficult to identify all the delinquency-learning processes in the open community; but the learning and unlearning processes in the treatment of offenders can at least be subjected to controlled experiment and detailed study. We shall deal briefly with some aspects of this balance of forces. These include, of course, not only institutional experience, but the problem of reintegration within the original community, and effective aftercare and rehabilitation in general.

One may ask first whether punishment can be expected to have much value in unlearning or rehabilitation. Most laboratory experiments suggest that punishment is of little use in the learning process; the positive rewarding of success leads to much more effective learning. Punishment may not succeed in doing more than warn the individual against embarking on certain types of behaviour, and may perhaps even help some non-offenders to avoid committing a crime; it may not, however, *help* the offender or show him the way out of his difficulties. But the results of laboratory studies have so far found little application in the controlled treatment of human

beings. There is a great need for a closer liaison between the laboratory worker and the practical therapist, and for controlled experiments based upon these findings. The technique for dealing with a
conflict of values, such as is found in the neurotic or psychiatric
case, may be fairly well understood; but changing antisocial values,
which have nevertheless been learnt by normal processes, probably
requires different methods, and is more difficult.

Little progress is likely unless account is taken of the great range of
motivation of delinquent acts. The sort of 'unlearning' required will
vary according to whether the motive of theft, for example, was a
desire to draw attention to oneself, a search for symbolic love, a
desire to overcome feelings of inferiority, or the need to attack
authority.

The delinquency-learning processes at work in the penal institution demonstrate in a concentrated but also distorted form many
of the forces at work in the outside community, and any attempt
to foster unlearning during detention must pay careful attention to
all these forces.

Imprisonment '. . . punishes the offender in a variety of ways
extending far beyond the simple fact of incarceration' (Sykes &
Messinger, 1960). He is rejected by society, and loses the ordinary
citizen's right to be trusted, and many features of his environment
emphasize this fact. His essential problem is to prevent rejection by
society from being converted into intolerable self-rejection. He
is cut off from his wife, family, or friends. There are not only the loss
of liberty and severely cramped conditions, but a level of material
existence which is reduced to bare subsistence, largely devoid of all
the elements of personal choice. Wives of prisoners may say that
'. . . he only has to sit there with everything provided, while I have
to pinch and scrape to support the children', but his knowledge of
this fact only emphasizes his devaluation. For many offenders the
outward signs of material possessions are especially necessary to
preserve their self-regard; they have none of the self-confidence of
the poor but proud. The sexual deprivation is not only a burden
in itself, but in those who have no overt homosexual tendencies
there may also be increased anxieties about homosexuality, and
(more important) it undermines the masculine self-concept which
bolsters morale in the free world which includes women – being
head of a house, or controller of children, etc. The lack of autonomy,

and submission to orders, revive a situation of childhood dependency, which his delinquent career may have been designed to avoid. Above all, 'the worst thing about prison is you have to live with other prisoners' (Sykes, 1956). Escape, not so much from prison as from other prisoners, is impossible. Aggressive or cunning fellow-prisoners are the cause of continued insecurity in maintaining one's social position, and in the fierce light of communal living no foibles or weaknesses escape detection (cf. also Sykes, 1958).

In this situation an inmate social system arises whose main function is 'to avoid the devastating psychological effects of internalizing and converting social rejection into self-rejection. In effect, it permits the inmate to reject his rejectors rather than himself' (McCorkle & Korn, 1954). This social system contributes most to those who have already experienced social rejection and have thus built up defences against it, and will find strongest support from those recidivists who have already made themselves independent of the values and supports of the wider community. Those who still have a large stake in this wider community find the social rejection difficult to bear, and have to make a difficult adaptation to the solace offered by the inmate social system.

A social code thus arises, of not co-operating with the authorities, of never betraying an inmate, of standing up for yourself firmly, of not interfering and not starting trouble, etc. Within this code there are of course 'deviants' – the strong-arm toughs who dominate, or the manœuvring 'merchants' who manipulate markets – but they strongly approve of the system themselves. All offenders, however, have to come to terms with this system. Schrag (1954) has shown that leaders tend to be those who have committed violent offences and are serving long sentences. G. Rose (1959), writing of a British borstal, differentiated anti-authority leaders, lieutenants, leader-aspirants who move up and down in success and failure, followers (followers from choice, or weak followers), independents (who include those mature boys who can maintain a balance of loyalty to staff and to fellow-inmates), and the rejected, who include friendship-seekers in whom no one will take an interest, and eccentrics who are regarded as strange by staff and boys. After release the leaders, lieutenants, and leader-aspirants tend to be reconvicted frequently, as do the rejected; the independents and some followers do best.

The custodial staff are also caught within this web. 'The keeper

H   99

of the keys is a prisoner too. By the time he retires, the custodian will have spent eight to fifteen years totally within prison walls' (McCorkle & Korn, 1954). He is greatly outnumbered, his personality characteristics will be studied carefully at very close quarters, and he is under constant threat of being outwitted by inmates. The small number of the staff, and the essential function of maintaining, if need be, security by physical force, require a strict discipline. But it is an army which never goes to war, but has to fight intangible psychological pressures. If in a strictly disciplined system the officer tries to cross the line between inmate and staff and develop what he wishes to be a helpful, personal relationship, the inmate tends to exploit this by special demands, by requesting a favour in return for a favour. When this has to be refused, a sense of 'betrayal' emerges on one side or the other, and the officer may be roused to an antagonism which did not exist before and which may be difficult to manage. The staff, whether custodial or workshop supervisors, find themselves obliged to strike a bargain or balance to obtain a smooth-running institution, which must often depend upon inmate collaboration. Work tends to be restricted by a strong tradition of minimal activity. The staff in daily contact with prisoners may find the pressure from their charges less difficult to bear than the pressure from the senior staff. The effect all too often is that the staff retreat into a routine attitude, mainly preoccupied, like some sergeants in the regular army, with making sure that they cannot be held responsible for what goes wrong. Even the outside visitor to a recidivist prison that is under antisocial tension may feel that he is manœuvred, passed around like a pawn, or deceived in minor ways by the staff; and this is the cynical image of the 'normal' well-adjusted world to which the prisoner is expected to give his allegiance.

The difficulties of prison life have been described in an extreme form, though there must be very few, if any, nations that could not produce examples of at least a few prisons to which this description would be partly applicable (Morris & Morris, 1963). The process occurs in spite of the goodwill and integrity of many of those who are locked within the system, and has indeed been observed in other institutions, such as psychiatric hospitals, as well as in prisons. There may be great variations in individual reaction, especially with regard to age. The younger the offender, the more likely will it be that the natural acceptance of some sort of adult control will lead to a more or less harmonious response to the organization of the school, though even in the institution for non-delinquent children, if strictly administered, one can perceive the common 'double standard' of the inmates, who pay genuine respect to an ideal type of conduct, but act according to a second standard laid down by whispered exchanges representing the most that can be reasonably expected of each other. Many institutions for selected adults, of course, avoid the worst of these features; a great deal presumably depends upon the proportion of severely disordered offenders in any institution.

Faced with an institution which, from its own inner necessity, seems doomed to drive its inmates to further social maladjustment, how is it possible to introduce a constructive process of 'unlearning'? In the free world, the psychotherapist who attempts to treat the gang member is perhaps faced with a similar problem. The answer, as many years of experience in several countries has shown, is not merely to introduce some psychiatrists and psychologists into prisons as we know them. Nor can a general humanitarian improvement in the conditions of imprisonment be expected to be effective in itself, however desirable it may be. As McCorkle, himself a psychotherapist and later a prison governor, says (McCorkle & Korn, 1954): 'Would the effect of specific conditions be to reduce the hostility, or would it require the inmate to find new outlets for it? Observations and experiences with the results of acceding to inmate pressure strongly suggest the latter. . . . The implications of this widespread psychological orientation for any treatment based chiefly on permissiveness and helping will become painfully obvious for any professional staff member who enters the prison with a missionary zeal and a determination to undo, by open-handed giving, the "evils of generations of prison corruption" . . . like some strange human hothouse, the prison has a way of developing a species of flowering "bleeding hearts" which put forth especially sticky and luxurious blossoms to ensnare the new professional. . . . The inmate social system throws a diversionary human screen of institutional "problem cases" around the professional staff member, eating up his time and misdirecting his efforts away from his proper target, the system itself.'

If this analysis suggested by McCorkle is correct, then the main influence upon the prisoner, the touchstone of his capacity to see himself as a problem and his hope of achieving adequate social relations on release, lie in his relations with other inmates. The main influence of the staff must be in affecting the general climate in which these relationships occur. Individual relations with staff or therapists will be effective only if they are compatible with this general climate.

In many countries, attempts are now made to prevent or oppose the system of criminal values fostered by the society of inmates, by bringing prisoners into much closer contact with the custodial staff in group discussions and group treatment. At the least, this ensures that the conflict in attitude is brought frankly into the open in an accepting atmosphere in which the merits or demerits of any attitudes can be reconsidered and discussed, and in time the emotions underlying these attitudes will find expression and exchange. Maintaining such contact imposes a great strain on the staff, for there can be no official institution rules about how junior staff are to respond to these shifting situations. It is only possible if the staff are selected and trained, and if they themselves meet regularly in groups of all sizes and at all administrative levels, so that they have the cohesion and confidence to offer an alternative to the inmate system. (Similar principles have been applied, in recent years, in dealing with the problems of staff–patient relationship in psychiatric hospitals – cf. Caudill, 1958; Greenblatt et al., 1955.)

The nature and function of such groups and contact-situations varies very widely, not only with the training and experience of the staff but especially with the age of the inmates and the degree to which they have been selected. Since group therapy has become such an acceptable term among penologists, it has been applied to almost all processes in institutions which aim to be therapeutic. From answers to questionnaires sent out to many institutions in 1950, McCorkle (1952) concluded that there were three basic approaches – the repressive-inspirational, the didactic, and the analytic. The first, or exhortation method, in McCorkle's view, '. . . uses the emotional appeal of the evangelistic revival meeting, combined with the commercial techniques of salesmanship to urge the participant to control himself by suppressing asocial or worrisome thoughts or wishes and, at the same time, find an inspiration in life – work, religion, etc.' The didactic method uses a class or lecture approach, with emphasis upon intellectual insight and verbal knowledge of psychological mechanisms. Analytically oriented treatment uses 'free association and intuitive interpretation of material presented by group members and urges the loosening of repression, and the conscious recognition and analysis of unconscious asocial wishes'. Some institutions reported recreational and occupational programmes as group therapy; as, indeed, they are, though not perhaps in this context. In many institutions there are work supervisors who are good therapists, aided by their neutrality in the hierarchy and the ability of a workgroup to tolerate periods of unhurried silence – action rather than words. The most widely accepted treatment used today is 'guided group interaction' (Slavson, 1951), in which the leader is active in the discussion and plays a supportive, guiding role throughout the course of the group's history. Although training in group leadership is important, it must necessarily follow that the personality of the leader gives a unique stamp to the group, and it is essential that he should work within the area in which he feels confident. Everyone learns partly from personal experience and partly from watching others learn. There are well-marked cultural differences in techniques of learning and techniques of self-criticism, in the tendency to verbalization or silence. One would expect groups in one country to take on a pedagogic or didactic flavour, in another to be highly verbalized and free. We all tend to approve a system which fits in with our cultural attitudes to how learning occurs. There is a need for more objective study of what is effective.

Techniques of treatment – group or individual – depend upon the selection of inmates. In the British psychopathic prison of Grendon, the staff at all levels conduct groups – officers, trade instructors, padres, psychologists, psychiatrists; these have a marked effect upon the climate of the institution. Inmates, however, are mentally abnormal (but not psychotic or defective) recidivists with fixed sentences, who volunteer to come to the institution and are only accepted after a selection process. Some cannot adjust to the climate of the institution and ask to be returned to the ordinary prison. In Denmark, on the other hand, at the Herstedvester medical institution, less responsive psychopathic prisoners are received without much selection for an indefinite period; this indefinite sentence is held to play an important role. Stürup (1952; 1959) describes his 'dynamic growth therapy' and the utilization of 'affective moments' (spontaneous catharsis) in changing a patient's point of view. Prolonged aftercare from the institution is possible. The machinery of intake and discharge has profound significance here, as in Atascadero, Vaccaville, or Patuxent institutions in the U.S.A. (Boslow *et al.*, 1959).

It goes without saying that a full programme of constructive and recreational activities in which the staff participate is needed. Many young offenders have a deep sense of inadequacy and ignorance in ordinary social and work situations. Even individual encouragement may at times make them worse, because it sharpens their anxious anticipation of failure, or because they are convinced that such praise or encouragement is sarcastic. In a group which succeeds in short-term projects, however, they feel the stirrings of achievement. Large-scale self-government is impossible because it denies the fact of compulsory detention, and tends to foster the aggressive leadership of the inmate culture; but opportunities for self-determination and planning, of practising and learning from the improvement in human relations, are needed. 'Some hardship or real lack in an institution is a great boon, provided it is within the community's capacity to correct; this, of course, was well known to all the pioneers but not, apparently, to the rich authorities who tend to supply their "problem" children on a lavish, material scale' (Scott, 1960b).

No one method is especially successful, nor can it be expected to be, in view of the vast range of personalities and problems. The psychiatrist oriented towards individual treatment naturally feels that we already have the psychiatric techniques to treat offenders – or a great many of them – provided society allowed the treatment to take place. But society's attitude, as this chapter may help to show, is, in a sense, part of the diagnosis. Such a view merely states the problem, but does not provide the solution. Individual psychotherapy in an ordinary prison often encounters this problem in an acute form.

The method of choice in relation to the type of offender has been discussed by Scott (1960a, b). Mackwood (1949), in a prison for adults, used the method of biographical reconstruction, enabling the offender to look at his past and future. Maxwell Jones *et al.* (1952; 1959) use group pressures in an open institution for psychopathic offenders or non-offenders to bring improved insight. Group-guided interaction (Weeks, 1958) at Highfields open institution for juveniles detained for a short period achieved considerable success, especially with the coloured delinquents within the predominantly white groups. Psychodrama (Moreno, 1946) and closed group analytical treatment in prison (Landers *et al.*, 1954) have also been used. The individual psychotherapy provided for juveniles in the PICO project (Adams S., 1961) demonstrated the importance of diagnosis in a well-controlled experiment. Those amenable to treatment (described as 'bright, verbal, anxious') were divided at random into treated and control groups, and the non-amenables were similarly treated or not treated at random. Untreated amenables and non-amenables were reconvicted at about the same rate over a period, and much more often than treated amenables. But, significantly, the treated non-amenables did worse than the untreated. This is one of several indications emerging from Californian studies, and first referred to by Grant and Grant (1959) in their exemplary study of naval detainees, that treatment wrongly applied may make the patient worse. For these more severely disordered offenders, forms of group-institutional treatment or the use of Stürup's moments of catharsis are perhaps needed.

Among the most pressing needs is that for genuinely experimental studies in the practical field, such as the above, and the interesting Provo study (Empey & Rabow, 1961) in which an experimental comparison is made of groups of delinquents sent either to a therapeutic community by day and going home at night, or kept on probation, or sent to a training school. There is also a need to bridge the large gap between experimental findings in the psychological laboratory and practical fieldwork. Fortunately, in the last ten years there have been signs of such communication.

One central problem on which laboratory studies of learning have thrown light has for too long been taken for granted, namely, whether punishment can be expected to influence behaviour favourably. Although many experiments have been carried out, the findings are confusing. 'It seems that, as a rule, punishment is a relatively inefficient way of changing behaviour, that its effect tends to diminish unless it is intense or is repeated; and that if it is intense, it may affect far more than the behaviour to which it was directed' (Gelder, 1965). In the penal field we may expect to reinforce the external controls upon some non-offenders, but the effect of penal methods upon the offender remains problematical and is undoubtedly very variable.

Among the new treatments stimulated by laboratory work are the various forms of 'behaviour therapy', though their origins date back to the earlier era of Janet (1925) and Meige and Feindel (1907), and the present theoretical foundations (Eysenck, 1964) may or may not be relevant to its practical effectiveness. Techniques of behaviour therapy in relation to the treatment of delinquents have recently been reviewed by Gelder (1965). They can be divided conveniently into those which aim to eradicate unwanted symptoms – so-called 'deconditioning' – and those which aim to encourage the development of aspects of behaviour which the patient lacks – so-called 'positive conditioning'. Techniques for deconditioning can in turn be divided into those which make use of anxiety relief, and others in which aversion is produced.

It is the aversion experiments that have been used with delinquents. They undoubtedly raise questions of medical ethics, since they involve the use by doctors of a punishment process; and, clearly, therapists must have a full insight into their own motives. In this case they consist of using unpleasant stimuli ('punishment') to suppress some form of behaviour which the patient wishes to be rid of, by drugs which induce nausea, or mild electric shocks. They have been used for some years in the treatment of alcoholism, and more recently, apparently with some success, in the treatment of various sexual aberrations, such as fetishism (Raymond, 1956), transvestism (Oswald, 1962; Smith, S. E., 1956; Pearce, 1963), and homosexuality (Freund, 1960). Deconditioning techniques, either systematic desensitization in imagination (Wolpe, 1958) or systematic desensitization by re-training (Meyer & Gelder, 1963; Gelder *et al.*, 1964)), have so far been used for the treatment of phobias, etc. and have not been extensively applied to delinquents, though exhibitionism has been treated in this way (Bond & Hutchison, 1960). The variability of these techniques suggests that important factors in their success are psychotherapy and the close relationship with the physician. On the whole, they are effective for isolated symptoms in those with good personality and few personal problems. Alcoholics with aggressive and disordered personalities, for example, are not suitable. It is indeed noteworthy that, on some occasions, these procedures have had paradoxical results: treatment aimed at a specific symptom has been relatively ineffective but has led to a noticeable improvement in social adjustment and general well-being, or reduction in the symptom has not led to a general improvement. The interplay of influences, and the psychological and physiological mechanisms involved, require careful study, and this is obviously far more important than theoretical controversies about the rationale of these forms of treatment.

The evident difficulties of providing an unlearning framework in institutions have encouraged the view that delinquents are better treated as far as possible at liberty, on probation, or with day attendance at institutions. The attitude towards deprivation of liberty is itself subject to great cultural differences. Tribal communities, accustomed to hunting or travelling great distances, tend to view imprisonment as a harsh penalty, worse than severe corporal punishment. Industrialized countries are influenced not only by the dangerousness of offenders but also, no doubt, by deeper cultural concepts of the place of liberty and the nature and needs of youth. At the cost of some exaggeration, one may say that in many States of the U.S.A. the child is allowed to commit many offences before coming to court, and is sent away to an institution for a relatively short time after repeated lapses. On reaching adult status, however, the offender is confined for long periods and, if he repeats his offences, may be quickly 'neutralized' by very long sentences of imprisonment. In England, the child is quickly brought before a court, and is sent away after only two or three offences for relatively long periods, which may be repeated in borstal training, with the idea that he will be re-educated or re-trained. By the age of twenty-three the offender may have spent five of six years in institutions. On his reaching adult status, however, society apparently despairs of further efforts: he is given a succession of quite short sentences unless he belongs to a very small minority of dangerous offenders. The first policy, presumably, has the risk of leaving children in a subcultural milieu for a long time – virtually until they become adults: and the concentration of adult long-term offenders in prison raises the many problems of institutional life discussed above. The second policy risks educating the child in a society of delinquents, with a concept of himself as a member of a criminal subculture; and the rapid succession of short terms of imprisonment as an adult, with virtually no parole or aftercare support on release, may go far to destroy his capacity for social adjustment. In local recidivist prisons, the atmosphere resembles that of a railway station or transit camp – 'that slaughterhouse of hope' (cf. Ahrenfeldt, 1958) – rather than a place of permanent residence. Other countries show variations upon these themes.

As international study and exchange increase, and perhaps under the uniform influence of urbanization, industrialization and rapid communication, the differences in such cultural attitudes are rapidly diminishing; and the willingness to make experimental studies of the value of particular treatments is steadily growing.

PART TWO

Chapter VII

ASPECTS OF THE WORLD SITUATION

Apart from discussing general principles and theories of culture in relation to delinquency, the Conference at Topeka aimed at comparing first-hand reports, from many parts of the world, of cultural influences and changes in the world today. In all countries patterns of delinquency are influenced by national, ethnic, or religious subgroups or by other minority groups; by migration, urbanization, industrialization, and other factors leading to rapid social change.

In the previous chapters we have discussed the general issues raised by the participants on the preliminary document, in many cases by reference to the situation in their own countries. After considering these issues, however, each participant was asked to comment upon the situation in his own country and to give specific examples of the varieties of cultural changes under discussion. One of the most important questions is whether these changes always have similar effects. Are there cases, for example, of urbanization and industrialization which have *not* led to an increase in delinquency? What differences are there between immigrants who have *not* encountered difficulties in a new country and those who have?

It is hardly surprising that answers to questions of this kind were not always available. Each participant, however, had particular comments to make about his own country. Many of these comments have been incorporated as specific examples in previous chapters, but there remain a number of questions and items of information which have not been mentioned. In the following pages these have been grouped in relation to particular countries, but it must not be supposed that they respectively summarize the remarks of any one participant; in many cases we have added other material within our own knowledge or suggested by the various participants. Many countries are, of course, not dealt with at all; the aim of the Conference was to be representative but, obviously, not comprehensive.

111

Australia

Australia has received some 11 per cent of its population since the Second World War. At first these immigrants were preponderantly from England, Holland, and Scandinavia; but more recently they have come from Southern, Central, and Eastern Europe. The government has many programmes to acclimatize them, such as 'Good Neighbour' Councils. Crime in the first generation of immigrants is lower than in the home-born. The use of knives in fights, which has been traditional among some immigrants in their country of origin, is not generally higher. The second generation, the children of immigrants, have not so far proved a problem as regards delinquency (cf. Victoria, State of, 1956). They readily adopt Australian customs and have not formed local delinquent groups or gangs. The Aborigines are protected as the inheritors of a valuable culture, and crime among them is insignificant.

Belgium

Belgium is a small country but, with nine million inhabitants, one of the most densely populated areas of the world. It has been heavily urbanized and industrialized for many decades. The incidence of juvenile delinquency (which is calculated up to the age of eighteen) rose sharply during the war, but recovered quickly afterwards and returned to pre-war levels (Racine, 1959; 1961). In the early nineteen-fifties there was a further upward trend. As in many countries, it is difficult to be sure how much of this increase was genuine, since it marked a new trend of the judiciary to concern itself with child welfare. The magistrates have been concerned to increase their welfare function, and the attitude of the police probably altered when they felt that they were required to *help* deprived young people, rather than to arrest and punish them. Nevertheless, there has probably been a real increase in delinquent behaviour. Institutions for delinquents are overcrowded, with waiting lists, which sometimes means that a young person has to be accommodated temporarily in jail; the judges claim to be overworked.

Increases in delinquency have occurred only in certain places; there is little in rural communities, where no doubt it is controlled by subcultural means. The labour force for the coal mines has been maintained by waves of immigrant workers. Before the war these were mainly Poles and Italians (many members of the British

Expeditionary Force to North-East France and Belgium in 1940 were startled to find public notices written in Polish), and successive waves have occurred since. Coalmining is unpopular with the Belgians themselves, and they discourage their children from taking it up. These immigrants are, in general, law-abiding communities, and the difficulties that arise are mainly over the issue of bringing in the whole family – a recurring problem in all countries, and one that receives very little political attention. But they seem to play a great part in precocious promiscuity among girls.

As in the Netherlands, visiting youths on holiday from Germany or Britain sometimes cause a good deal of difficulty – stealing cars, committing sex offences, etc. There have been very few teenage riots.

Traffic offences, shoplifting, and stealing cars (which is not thought of as stealing) have increased, as in many countries. There has also been some increase in homosexual prostitution, which is relatively new. It is not confined to big cities and cafés, but is found in mining areas and elsewhere.

There has been a considerable increase in juvenile gangs, usually of boys of seventeen or eighteen but including any age from fourteen to twenty-five. The leaders and deputies are not always the oldest. They commit some property offences, but are also involved in sexual molestation or aggressive offences, especially against people of different class or language, or the police. They are found not only in large cities but also in small towns, based upon some café or dance-hall. They show Americanized influences and call themselves (in English) the Wild Cats or Black Cats and model themselves upon James Dean or Elvis Presley. Members of gangs come from a working-class background, but not from poverty-stricken or problem families in any extreme sense. They have little connection with adults, except with some disreputable ones such as homosexual prostitutes or delinquent characters. Generally they are of the *blouson noir* type, but there are also reported to be a few upper-class gangs – *blousons dorés*.

One feature is their conventionality and lack of inventiveness. They do not emulate singing stars of their own choice, but follow current popular models. The twenty-five-year-old members remain very juvenile in both outlook and mentality.

Canada

With regard to Canada, our informants suggested that there was a considerable increase in organized types of crime. Some 56 per cent of those convicted of crime are in the age group 16–25. Among these there are said to be many who have little interest except to live by crime. Although many do not fully realize it, they are part of a system of organized crime; receiving, for example, regular consignments of stolen goods for resale without knowing where they came from, but being paid regularly. This pay is large enough to give them little incentive to lead an honest life. Few juveniles commit crimes on their own over a prolonged period of time; these are usually organized and planned for them. At the age of 25–30, they are far less frequently arrested, but this may only be because they hand over the simpler jobs (e.g. stealing certain types of car in the street) to younger boys and graduate to the part of the network that is relatively free from arrest. This, in turn, may only mean that they are considered too unreliable to be trusted with the organization of rackets, and have to depend more and more on their own initiative and boldness. Those who are concerned with buying stolen goods will not accept unreliable and inexperienced providers and will deal only with quiet, discreet accomplices.

An increasing number of middle-class boys are involved in habitual delinquency. A number of profitable rackets are often found to be connected with those who have been to high school or college. It may start as a joke or episode of excitement but turn out to be so profitable that boys continue with it. The difference between urban and rural crime is decreasing – a gang may be composed of two city boys and two who live in the country near by. Similarly, the meeting-places for these groups are no longer the pool-rooms and street corners, but country clubs, or night clubs, parks, or squares in the centre of the city.

When seen in institutions, many delinquents are incompetent, inadequate – although intelligent – youths who are organized and used by those better socialized than themselves. There is little real cohesion in the groups they form; these tend to be groups of passive boys who could never gain acceptance in more positive groups. Similarly, riots are not organized; they are merely contagious. Absconding, also, is rarely organized: boys run away in groups only because they are too fearful to take any step alone. The disturbance of and the deviation from the socialization process are a cardinal feature; these are not structured gangs, but groups of helpless individuals clinging together for support. Such groups, in fact, tend to show a disintegration of any kind of social pattern (cf. Lavallée & Mailloux, 1964; Mailloux & Lavallée, 1960; 1962).

Immigration to Canada has been on a large scale, and very successful. Immigrants have been selected, are quite often skilled, and have not been despised by the indigenous population. They have been directed to the areas where their work is needed, and told with some accuracy what to expect, so that there is little disappointment or disillusionment. The rate of delinquency and crime among them has been remarkably low.

Colombia

In Colombia the situation has been dominated by the concept of *violencia* – the special political type of homicide which started fifteen years ago and has been responsible for some quarter of a million deaths: whole villages are attacked by roving bands who later become victims of massive reprisals, etc. The general acceptance of this killing is unique. (Saavedra & Rave, 1963. See pages 70–71 above). There are large numbers of abandoned children, many of whom have seen their parents killed before their eyes. They have an embittered and hostile attitude to almost any sort of organization and are ready to be aggressive in any situation. Some five hundred children a year disappear – if they are crippled, it is assumed that they have been taken to the cities to help with begging. For many children basic needs for survival are not provided; there is widespread begging, passing easily to aggression and stealing. It has been said that 'one cannot impose the law on an empty stomach'. Re-education for these children is only provided at the rate of 1 peso for every 66 pesos spent on repression. The modern generation is struggling to make headway with these difficulties, with some success (cf. also Fandiño, 1962; Guzman, 1962).

Israel

Israel is unique from a demographic point of view. It forms a laboratory for the study of immigration problems; but the small size of its population, the high proportion of social scientists and other trained observers, and the relatively high degree of social cohesion, must make the conditions of immigrants very different from those who affected the unplanned migrations in other countries and epochs.

The flow of immigrants into Palestine, and the later State of Israel, has been almost continuous, though with marked fluctuations, since the beginning of the century. At the creation of the State of Israel in 1948, the Jewish community in Palestine (the Yishuv) numbered about 650,000; but the majority of these were fairly recent immigrants. 'The Yishuv . . . was not merely an immigrant absorbing community. . . . It was also a community which immigrants had created. The time span between the establishment of its first institutional outlines and the influx of waves of immigrants was very short . . . and its institutional structure was in continuous formation and development while these various waves were entering' (Eisenstadt, 1954). Three-quarters of the pre-1948 immigrants were of European origin; nearly one-half of these were from Poland. Immigration was at a low level from 1939 to 1948, but from 1948 to 1958 nearly 900,000 new immigrants arrived – 30 per cent from Asia (mainly Iran), 44 per cent from Europe (especially Poland and Rumania), and 25 per cent from Africa (Tunis, Algeria, Morocco, etc.), especially in the later stages. The original 'receiving' community of 1948, mainly European, was, therefore, outnumbered by new arrivals, of which more than half were Asian or African in origin.

Reifen (1960) states that, in recent years, immigrant Jews originating from Asia, the Near and Middle East, and North Africa have increased numerically to about half of the population. Cultural conflict has resulted from transplantation into a competitive, urbanized and industrialized, 'Western' type of society. The process of culture change is most marked in Oriental communities, where negative repercussions are particularly felt: over 80 per cent of juvenile delinquents are of Eastern origin. Richelle et al. (1957) have given a good account of the social, cultural, educational, and psychological background of young North African Jews (mainly from Morocco), and the problems encountered by them after immigration into Israel. They point out that, in recent years, increasing attention has been given by the Israeli Government to the needs of children originating from Asian countries and from

116

North Africa, so that these constituted 75 per cent of the 12,500 young immigrants, aged 13–17 years, who were taken under the care of the Aliyat Hanoar in 1957.

The criminal behaviour of immigrants in Israel has been described by Shoham (1962). Between 1953 and 1957 the 60 per cent of the population who were adult immigrants comprised 67 per cent of the offenders, a ratio of 'new' to 'old' inhabitants of 10 to 7·5. There was a considerable difference, however, in the incidence of criminality by immigrants of different origins. For serious offences per 1,000 immigrants this was, in 1957, 13 from Africa, 10 from Asia, and 5 from Europe or America. Migrants from Africa were mainly from the 'Moghrebite' communities in North Africa with very different cultural and educational standards from those of Asiatic Jews. There was also a difference in type of offence according to ethnic origin – 40 per cent of African Jews being convicted of offences against the person, arson, and damage to property, as compared with 32 per cent of European Jews.

American studies, however, have tended to show that the main culture conflict with respect to crime and immigration arises with the second generation. The native-born of immigrant parents, or those who immigrated at a very young age, are the most prone to suffer. The conduct norms of the immigrants differ from those of the receiving country; and the process of integration may shatter the social and economic status of the head of the family. 'The oriental Jewish father, however poor he may be, is always the omnipotent paterfamilias. But when he comes to Israel, the different social set-up may prevent him from fully exercising his former status, he may be given a job not to his liking, and the different living conditions may shatter his previous convictions and leave him in a state of confusion in which he cannot exercise proper control over his family. The youngster may also realize that his father is not the omnipotent patriarch he was supposed to be, and sometimes when he comes home from school he may see his father signing a document with his ink-stained thumb' (Shoham, 1962). These factors may persuade the child to throw in his lot with his contemporaries in the 'street culture', a tendency which, in any case, has similarly been evident in a number of other countries.

Juvenile delinquency in Israel has risen steadily from 1949 to 1959 from 0·68 per cent of the relevant age group to 1·32 per cent.

The rates for immigrant delinquents were, however, 311 per 100,000 in 1958, compared with 188 for the total juvenile population. Immigrants* have larger families than the 'old' inhabitants, but this is not thought to explain altogether the difference in delinquency rate, which is, for 1957 and 1958, in the ratio of 10 'new' to 6 'old' residents. It is difficult to disentangle the various factors which may possibly be involved, but the highest rates occur in areas, such as parts of Haifa, which are almost totally inhabited by immigrants. The highest rate of all is found in the rural area around Jerusalem, which is entirely immigrant, where the rate in 1957 was 455, compared with 189 in Jerusalem city. The Agranat Committee on Juvenile Delinquency (1956) concluded that whether 'new' or 'old', the oriental Jews produced a great preponderance of delinquency, and that 'the process of social and cultural integration of the oriental immigrant boy is seemingly accompanied by cultural and external conflicts which result inter alia in delinquency'. If not helped to integrate, he may develop a feeling of being the subject of discrimination and will become increasingly maladjusted as time goes by. The European boy may have initial difficulties but these are, as a general rule, gradually overcome. The Committee also noted that 'cultural differences (i.e. oriental-European) have a greater causal significance than the sheer fact of immigration'.

As Shoham (1962) points out, in the causation of culture conflict, 'immigration or ethnic differences are only two aspects of the same problem', and he suggests that the conflict is liable to be greater when immigrants arrive together from *many*, rather than from only one or two different, cultures.

Shoham and Hovav (1964) have also investigated the problems of delinquency among the middle- and upper-class youth (the 'B'nei-Tovim'). These were defined as either having parents in white-collar jobs, with superior incomes and living in better residential areas, or being in higher education themselves, or both. Among over one thousand delinquents, 29 per cent were 'middle and upper class' by these criteria, 53 per cent lower class, and the remainder unclassifiable. Immigration patterns were immediately apparent, for 66 per cent of the B'nei-Tovim boys came from families who were already in Israel in 1948, as compared with 53 per cent of

* Native-born children of immigrants cannot be distinguished, in the available statistics, from those who immigrated at a very early age.

the lower class: moreover, 66 per cent of the B'nei-Tovim were Ashkenazi Jews (from Europe), while 80 per cent of the lower class were oriental (from the former Turkish Empire) or Sephardic Jews (originally from Spain). Of the delinquents themselves, 70 per cent of the B'nei-Tovim, but only 42 lower class, had been born in Israel.

The B'nei-Tovim tended to commit offences of vandalism and pointless aggression and 'living in the moment' offences to satisfy immediate needs. They were more often first offenders only, and were more leniently treated on the first offence though not subsequently. Their homes had less often been broken, and their parents were less unstable or passive. A large number of the B'nei-Tovim displayed a negativistic, defiant, and rebellious attitude towards society, as reflected in their comments on their offences, but many others showed a strong sense of guilt. They had fewer previous convictions and subsequently abandoned crime more rapidly. At the age of fourteen, middle-class delinquents actually were in the majority, while the lower-class, with repeated offences, predominated at fifteen or sixteen.

The B'nei-Tovim thus have many characteristics of the middle-class delinquent in all countries, but in Israel there are many crosscurrents. Though they come from more stable and privileged homes, they are involved in adolescence in a conflict of values which arises perhaps from cultural factors with uncertainty about themselves and, especially, uncertainty about their parents. The fact that 75 per cent of the population are new immigrants, and that the 'receiving' community is in the minority, must expose the parents to changing standards, and uncertainty. – (Cf. also works marked * in Bibliography.)

Italy

In Italy juvenile delinquency has been decreasing for some years, following an increase soon after the war. There is considerable internal migration from the rural South to the industrial centres of Turin, Milan, and Genoa, but this has not been accompanied by a very noticeable increase in delinquency in those centres. There has also been a migration to Rome and here, too, the increase in juvenile delinquency has been negligible – the population has risen by 10 per cent and delinquency by only 4 per cent. Gangs are rare in Italy, except in certain cities such as Naples and Palermo, where they have a long tradition (cf. Franchini & Introna, 1961).

Much may depend upon the age and circumstances of the migrant. Where, as in Italy, a father migrates with his family to a new and better job in another part of the country, his moral and physical authority in the family is maintained, especially if adequate social circumstances are guaranteed. Many other migrants – for example, the Italians themselves when emigrating to other countries (Racine, 1959, 1961) and the Irish, Jamaicans, or Indians coming to England – come alone at first and only later bring their families, and there may be difficulties with housing, etc. In Israel, the family may come as a whole, but the father may rapidly lose authority because his standard of education is lower than that soon achieved by his sons.

Italy, nevertheless, contains within its culture the largest and most successful criminal organization in Europe – the Mafia (see pages 64–65). It is still a matter of speculation as to how far the Mafia has supplied the cohesion in the criminal underworld of the United States, and how much organized international crime (in drug-trafficking, etc.) has followed the compulsory repatriation to Italy of some well-known gangsters (Lewis, 1964; cf. Allen, 1962).

Somewhat ironically, after the considerable, and largely successful, efforts of Mussolini to stamp out this organization, it reappeared in strength during and after the war, principally as a result of the very skilled use made of the *mafiosi* by the Americans during the campaign in Sicily (Lewis, 1964). In recent years, attempts have once again been made by the Italian government to introduce suitable measures for the eradication of this traditionally, socio-culturally deeply rooted institution (Nat. Council on Crime & Delinquency, 1963; Puleo, 1962).

Japan

Japan is undergoing very rapid social change. The rate of economic growth is exceptionally high – three times that of such a rapidly growing country as the United States. Social organization, which used to be supported by complex 'extended' family units and low social mobility, is changing rapidly, with the emergence of the Western type of 'nuclear' family, comprising only parents and children, and with increased social mobility. The traditional extended family absorbed more delinquent conduct without making it

120

public and better insulated its members from delinquency than does the modern nuclear family. Moreover, traditional Japanese houses were constructed in such a fashion that their protection necessitated one member of the family always being at home; the modern apartment, often empty for much of the day, is easily entered by thieves.

The young are under great pressure to achieve high-school status and a college or technological education. Even physically, there are differences between the generations; the youths being perceptibly taller than the adults, as in some European countries. The suicide rate is exceptionally high among Japanese youth (cf. Iga, 1961). The introduction of legalized abortion has practically abolished 'illegal' abortions (only one such case was officially reported in 1960 (Ministry of Justice, 1963)). Statistics are, therefore, not comparable with those of most other countries.

Excluding traffic offences which, as elsewhere, continue to mount, there has not been an increase in total crime. Since 1956 adult crime has tended to diminish but there has been a rapid increase in juvenile delinquency from 1956–60, with some stabilization in 1962 and 1963, and a further increase in 1964. Wilson and Wilson (1964) reported recently that offences under the penal code of the age group 10–20, which were 3·2 per 1,000 of the relevant age group in 1939 to 1940, rose to 7·6 per 1,000 in 1947 to 1950, and 9·6 per cent in 1960 – an increase which seems about the same as that occurring in England. After 1961, however, the increase in Japan appears to have levelled out.

The peak age for offences in Japan appears to be later than in many other countries – at about nineteen (15·7 per 1,000 in the group 18–20), but comparisons, as always, are difficult, since under the age of fourteen a great many cases of delinquency are not dealt with by the Family Court, but are handled administratively under the Child Welfare Law by Child Guidance Centres. This accounts in part for the low level of recorded delinquency from ten to fourteen years. After sixteen, particularly serious cases can be handed over to the Public Prosecutor, but this occurs in only 9 per cent of cases.

According to the Japanese Government's White Paper on Crime (Ministry of Justice, 1963), 'Seven characteristics of juvenile crime have been observed. These are (1) commission of more serious types of offences; (2) increase in the incidence of crime committed by groups; (3) increase in juvenile recidivism; (4) increase in the incidence of crime committed by the low-teenage group; (5) increase in crime committed by students; (6) increase in the numbers of juvenile offenders from middle-class families; and (7) a concentration of juvenile crime in the big city.'

While the increase in general delinquency seems to correspond, for example, with the English post-war pattern, there is a distinctly higher proportion of crimes of violence in Japan – 25 per cent compared with 8 per cent in England. Rape, too, is relatively frequent in Japan, 2·2 per cent of all penal juvenile offences in Japan in 1960 compared, for example, with 0·1 per cent in England. Rape, however, is subject to very variable definition; and since there are many more non-indictable offences (excluding motoring offences) by juveniles in England, many of which are minor aggressive offences, it may be that there is not such a great difference.

Apart from increased violence, there is an increase in group activity, and an involvement of young people in protection rackets and prostitution organizations. One of the most marked events was the spread in the use of amphetamine stimulants among teenagers, to which we have already referred (Naka, 1956; Foran, 1962). This anticipated a similar wave of misuse in England. After control legislation had been passed in Japan, the teenagers seem to have taken to the misuse of barbiturate sedatives, and it is a question of interest whether in England a similar movement will take place after the control legislation of 1964. Barbiturates are in such widespread use for general therapeutic purposes that their control is difficult, and there must be some anxiety whether the same development will occur in England.

De Vos and Mizushima (1960; 1962) also point out that Koreans in Japan are a socially and economically underprivileged minority group. There is a stereotype in Japan that they are responsible for much delinquency and crime. The Korean minority has, in fact, a high delinquency rate and is more prone to the use of drugs: they show 'many of the signs of American minority groups in respect to delinquent patterns' (De Vos & Mizushima, 1962).

Japanese authorities seem to make little distinction between the liability of boys and girls to be brought before the courts (Wilson & Wilson, 1964). Nevertheless, offences by females, consisting mainly of theft, seem to have remained constant while the boys' offences have increased, so that the sex ratio has declined from 1 girl to 10 boys, to 1 girl to 17 boys.

When asked about the causes of the increase in delinquency, Judge Morita (Wilson & Wilson, 1964) emphasized social tension, particularly between the generations, as the main factor. Under this term he included social mobility, cultural differences, differences in ways of spending money, and 'fanatical religion' in the older generation. It is significant that over one-third of the juvenile delinquency in Tokyo is attributable to young people who have left their homes elsewhere in the country and come to Tokyo, either with their parents' consent (students and apprentices), or by 'elopement'. The usual area studies show that homes of delinquents are scattered fairly equally all over the city: studies of the place of commission of delinquent acts reveal a massive concentration around the main railway stations and entertainment areas (cf. also De Vos & Mizushima, 1959; 1960; 1962).

Mauritius

The island of Mauritius is also one of the most densely populated areas in the world, and of great interest from a cultural standpoint because of the well-marked ethnic groupings.

The island was first thoroughly colonized by the French, who introduced the staple trade of the island (sugar production) and who, under a succession of distinguished Governors, built up a French land-owing aristocracy. When the island was ceded to Britain in 1814 the rights and privileges of this group were guaranteed, and they preserve the cultural features of a proud ruling class. The young men were promiscuous with other islanders but not with the French girls, and they were rarely brought to court for any offences which they may have committed. They might obstruct the police and considered themselves entitled to take the law into their own hands in minor ways. Assaults are, however, more frequently reported to the police today. When slavery was abolished in 1835, labour on the plantation was provided by imported Indian indentured workers. They suffered much exploitation in the nineteenth century, necessitating British Government inquiries, but gradually took over most of the business and trade, as well as some of the land. The Hindus have recently achieved political control. Later, there was an influx of Chinese.

The 'mixed' population of French-African half-castes, etc., the most delinquent section of the population, live mainly in the cities

123

and are caught between the political power of the Indians and the economic power of the French. Assaults and woundings are common offences. Delinquency in the age group 10–21 rose from 30 per 10,000 to 46 per 10,000 in 1962–3. Taking hashish or marihuana was formerly confined to the Indians but has spread to the mixed population. With them, illegitimacy, broken homes, truancy, and common-law marriages of an ephemeral kind are very common.

Among the girls, culturally accepted stealing by servants is quite common and takes on almost compulsive features. Even when servants are given all the food they need, they still feel they must exercise their traditional right to steal, and will take surplus food quite unnecessarily.

The Hindus, with the assumption of political power and greater security, have become less delinquent. Their crime rate fell from 25 per 10,000 in 1960 to 20 per 10,000 in 1963. The Muslim minority among the Indians, however, have become increasingly insecure, and their delinquency rose between 1960 and 1963 from 20 per 10,000 to 28 per 10,000. Muslims tend to be promiscuous and show great concern for their potency.

There were no criminal gangs until 1963, but, at that time, following the showing of films about *blousons noirs*, a certain number of teenage gangs appeared, whose members wore black jackets, etc. Some adult recidivists organized some of the shopbreaking expeditions. In 1964, a French psychopath organized a gang of recidivists who carried out quite dangerous robberies and housebreakings. No one could catch them, but the local population established a squad of vigilantes who finally killed one of the gang. Although twenty people were prosecuted for this killing, all were acquitted. There was also an incident of hooliganism when a gang of teenagers caused such trouble in a certain village that one could not stop there in a car without risk of damage. This group had detached themselves from the usual group organizations in the community, but they banded together and took as their symbol British B.S.A. air-rifles with which they caused annoyance. The choice of a symbol of group activity from outside the traditional culture is of some interest.

The Netherlands

After the war there was some increase in the amount of violence accompanying theft, which was found among both those who had been collaborators *and* those who had been members of the resistance. Memories of the Underground warfare do not incline any Dutch people to suppose that excessive violence is confined to Colombia!

There was no ethnic problem until after the war, when the population of Amboina in the Netherlands East Indies, who were Christians and had remained loyal to the Dutch, were evacuated to the Netherlands. The repatriated Indo-Dutch population also caused some difficulties. The immigrants from the Netherlands West Indies and Surinam who came to the Netherlands also received very bad publicity – their origin was always mentioned when one of them committed an offence, but statistically they have not proved to be proportionally more delinquent (cf. Pronk, 1961). After the Hungarian insurrection the Netherlands agreed to accept 10,000 Hungarians; it has been very difficult to resettle them. One local form of crime, which also occurs in Belgium, is that German youths, who are apparently law-abiding at home, come for holidays or day excursions and give a rise to a good deal of thoughtless hooliganism.

Some 80–90 per cent of delinquency in Holland is committed in groups. As in several other countries of Western Europe, there has been much discussion of the apparent loosening or weakening of roles in the community – adolescents are less differentiated, or more uncertain, in their roles in relation to adults. In addition, boys and girls seem inclined to confuse or reverse sex-role differences, the boys wearing long hair and the girls wearing trousers, high boots, and other forms of masculine apparel. This phenomenon, as is well known, has become widespread in recent years in Western countries; and, according to a press report (November 1964), increasing numbers of Swedish teenage boys are taking to lipstick, face powder, and wearing bows in their long, wavy hair – ('borrowing' these articles from their sisters) – apparently with the approval of their girl friends.

*Nigeria**

Nigeria is beginning to show an increase in delinquency. The extended family system reduces not only delinquency, but also the extent to which it is reported; but this system is breaking down in the cities. Adolescents drift to the towns and are exposed to new pressures. There are none of the cultural ties and controls that they

* For a report on the former *French* West African territories, see pp. 154–8.

are used to; some arrive with nowhere to go and no job. There is little employment for young people, so that resettlement after release from an institution is difficult. When boys are sent to an approved school there is no tendency to abscond because they welcome the security of institutionalization. For all these reasons a considerable increase in delinquency may be expected in the future.

In Ibadan, with a population of half a million, stealing is commoner than minor forms of violence, but this proportion is reversed in the smaller towns. Many more children are picked up and sent home from the larger cities. The sex distribution among delinquents is 88 boys to 12 girls.

Parents exert considerable pressure on their children to make educational progress. Teachers soon get impatient with children who do not make rapid progress, but there are few facilities for backward children or those who need special treatment, so that educational failure is a frequent cause of maladjustment. As discussed earlier, education is free, but school attendance voluntary; so that a very rapid differentiation of the population is taking place into educationally determined strata, reflecting not only the talents of the children but even more the outlook and ambitions of the parents. Benzedrine is sometimes used to improve school-work, as well as out of the usual teenage interest, and homeless children are readily induced to become messengers in the black market in amphetamines and marihuana.

The culture of East and West Nigeria has many similarities, but in the Northern area, which is still very feudal, and is predominantly Moslem, delinquents tend to be culturally 'contained' and there are few facilities either for detecting or for reporting offences.

In cases studied, there are more delinquents from monogamous than polygamous homes, relative to their distribution in the community. But information derived from children is not always correct and much depends upon the type of polygamy. Very often a man makes a first marriage when quite young, the marriage being arranged by the family. Some years later, the first wife may herself suggest that the husband should get a younger woman for a second wife, and in such cases there are likely to be quite good relations between several women in the house. When the husband marries again without the agreement of the other wives, there may naturally be much tension. Some marriages are reported by the children as monogamous, when in fact there is only one woman at home in what was once a polygamous family.

There is usually sufficient food, and stealing for survival is not at all common. An unusual feature is that only 22 per cent of delinquents commit their offences in company with others.

Poland

Unfortunately, none of those attending the Topeka Conference was able to give a first-hand account of juvenile delinquency in Poland. A valuable unpublished paper by Dr Jerzy Jasinski (1962) and reports edited by Professor Batawia (1960–4) are, however, available. Juveniles are defined as those under the age of seventeen, and though there is no official minimum age, it has been a common practice since about 1954 not to sentence to educational training children who have not completed their tenth year.

Juvenile delinquency has increased between 1951 and 1964 from about 4·6 per 1,000 to 6·5 per 1,000, but annual fluctuations have been considerable and a number of factors, including alteration in police practice, etc., raise doubts about the exact trend, especially in the young adults of 17–20 years. Figures for 1962, however, by age group, show an increased rate of delinquency for each year of life up to a peak age of nineteen, when delinquency is three to four times the rate at the age of twelve or thirteen. About 10 boys to 1 girl are convicted in the younger age group, but only 7 to 1 at the age of nineteen, which is also the peak age for crime by girls.

The vast majority of crimes by young boys are property offences, but offences 'against life and health', though rarely of a serious kind, become increasingly common with advancing age, so that at the peak age of nineteen they account for 24·6 per cent of all offences. It is not known how far the excessive drinking reported in recent years among youths in Poland, as in Czechoslovakia (Sieliczka, 1961; Mecír, 1961), contributes to this high rate of violent offences. In 1960, 77·6 per cent of the juveniles came from intact homes, 17·6 per cent had only a mother, and 3·5 per cent only a father, and 1·1 per cent were orphans – a much lower incidence of broken homes than in 1953. A relatively high proportion of offences (34–39 per cent) were committed by boys with two or more companions, and between 20–25 per cent of all the juveniles convicted were not attending school or working at the time.

Jasinski has paid much attention to the possible effects of internal migration, urbanization, and industrialization on juvenile and young adult delinquency. Poland has had to deal with two internal migrations in recent years. First, there was the redistribution of population after the devastation by war (in the North-west, only about 3 per cent of the present population lived there before the war, as compared with 95 per cent in the Central and Eastern provinces). Second, there has been a movement toward centres of industrialization. Juvenile and young adult delinquency has usually been highest in those provinces where the shift of population following the Second World War has been the greatest, and where (in the period from 1952 to 1957) the influx has been greatest.

The migrations have been associated with many processes, such as increasing industrialization and urbanization. The districts with the highest rates of juvenile delinquency have been those with the largest proportion of their population 'employed outside agriculture' (i.e. industrialized); they are also districts where the majority live in cities and where the speed of urban growth has been highest.

Puerto Rico

Puerto Rico, an island with some two and a half million inhabitants, presents many problems of great social interest. It is undergoing a more rapid social change than almost any other modern society. It has the second highest average income in Latin America, being surpassed only by Venezuela, with the important difference, however, that in Puerto Rico the taxation system distributes the wealth widely, whereas in Venezuela, 95 per cent of the national income is concentrated in the hands of 5 per cent of the population.

The population of Puerto Rico is expanding very rapidly – 50 per cent of the population are under the age of twenty-one. They can come and go to the United States without restriction, and when in New York, where they tend to concentrate, they can go on relief at once. Some sixty thousand have left home for the United States in certain years. At present, however, re-immigration is increasing, and the migration balance is negative. Industrialization and urbanization are making rapid strides, and the tourist trade is assuming great importance.

Crime in Puerto Rico has increased considerably in the past few years. The most recent figures show that between 1957 and 1962 the adult proportion of the convicted grew by 17·3 per cent. Police intervention for crimes committed by juveniles during 1962 and 1963 increased 13·7 per cent over the preceding year.

These social changes, which are usually regarded as predisposing to a sharp increase in delinquency, have been intensified by certain special features of migration. Many delinquent patterns of conduct are brought back from New York by returning migrants. In the last five years, for example, a group of 12,000 young narcotic addicts has emerged, largely composed of those who learnt the habit in the United States. Gang behaviour is unusual among the indigenous population of the island but has also increased, chiefly among the youths returning from the United States; the same is true of violent crime, which is unusual in the local population and still does not occur on a great scale. Dramatic suicides are a special feature – in one month of a recent year there were fourteen suicides who soaked themselves in petrol and set it on fire.

Migration causes other cultural problems. Girls in Puerto Rico are strictly chaperoned, in the Spanish tradition. If this custom is abandoned on going to New York, they may come to be regarded on return by the neighbours and by boys as 'loose girls', and so become exposed to special temptation. Puerto Ricans who return home are not necessarily those who have failed to succeed in New York; but when they return with new skills, they may not find employment. Children who go to New York when young suffer to some extent in the schools because they do not speak English, although trials of special tuition are being made. Later, when they return to Puerto Rico, they are looked down on because they cannot speak Spanish, and it has recently become necessary to provide Spanish lessons for the returned migrant!

In Puerto Rico, as in some of the rural areas of Southern Italy, conditions of nutrition and childbirth are slow to improve in spite of new medical and social services. In such areas, subnormal or birth-injured children may swell the ranks of delinquents. Organic factors may play a relatively large part in the causation of delinquency.

Scandinavia

Denmark is a homogeneous society, almost entirely North European in ethnic origin and Protestant in religion, though religion does not play a forceful part in the culture. There is only one small minority group of Germans near the border and, though they caused trouble by collaborating with the enemy during the Second World War, they have not contributed much to delinquency either before or after that time. The social organization is that of a 'welfare society', and there has been no conspicuous increase in delinquency (Christiansen, 1959; 1960), in contrast to Sweden and Norway, which many obervers would suppose to have many cultural similarities.

In Sweden there has not only been an increase in delinquency, but the development of some teenage violence and rioting which has caused some concern (Christiansen, 1960). In Norway, there has been an appreciable increase in juvenile delinquency, which in 1960 was 70 per cent higher than in 1950 (Norwegian Committee, 1960); but there have been only a few serious youth riots. As Christiansen (1960) observes: 'A thorough study of these striking differences in the trend of juvenile and youthful criminality in countries which are closely related from a socio-cultural point of view, would be of very great interest. Such a study has been planned for the Scandinavian countries. . . .' It may be hoped that with the establishment, in 1962, of a Scandinavian Research Council for Criminology, on the initiative of the governments of Denmark, Finland, Norway, and Sweden, this important cross-cultural study will be successfully completed, but the difficulties in establishing similar definitions and statistical bases, even in such relatively homogeneous areas, demonstrate the problems referred to in the first chapter.

In Denmark, 8 per cent of the population are convicted some time in their lives, 6 per cent before the age of twenty-five, the remaining 2 per cent by those of all ages over twenty-five. Between 1939 and 1943, crime increased – almost doubled – and there was a three- or fourfold increase in the population of the penal institutions, but this subsided after the war.

Christiansen (1964) has examined the question of a Danish 'delinquent generation' by methods similar to those of Wilkins (1960). He found that children born between 1927 and 1932 had a higher rate of delinquency than the expected level of a long period; between 1932 and 1939 the incidence was below the expected level. The highest crime rate was registered for children born during the period 1939–43, the excess rate being about 30 per cent. Wilkins found that the excess crime rate in England occurred in those children who were four or five years old during the war years, and it might seem strange that in Denmark the greatest excess was in children who were four or five in 1943–8. Christiansen (1955; 1964) points out, however, that before 1943 the German occupation did not have a great impact upon social life. On 29th August, 1943 the official government policy of negotiation and collaboration was definitely abandoned; from this date, Denmark was in a state of war with Germany or in a comparable state of emergency. General strikes occurred during the summer of 1943; the persecution of the Jews began in October 1943; only 6 of the 435 patriots executed by the Germans lost their lives before August 1943; the organization of the army of the resistance movement began in the autumn of 1943; 45 per cent of the quislings and 60 per cent of *non*-Nazi traitors detected were recruited in the last sixteen months of the war. There were many objective signs that the serious social dislocation of war began in 1943, with the main emphasis on the period from 1942 to 1945.

In other fields of delinquency there are marked differences in the Scandinavian countries. Arrests for drunkenness in Helsinki and Oslo are nine times as high as in Denmark, and there are three or four times as many arrests in Stockholm and Oslo generally as in Copenhagen. Denmark has much more liberal laws regulating the use of alcoholic drinks than the other Scandinavian countries. Which may be the cause and which the effect is always a delicate matter in evaluating the significance of such statistics.

One of the most interesting studies of group delinquency has been made by a Norwegian criminologist, Sveri (1960). He found that offences committed by groups of four or more children were at their maximum at eight or nine, and very few at this age were committed by solitary offenders. After the age of sixteen, however, solitary offenders began to predominate and groups of four or more became increasingly rare after eighteen.

Homicide is rare in Denmark, but suicide is exceptionally high. The abolition of the death penalty many years ago has had the result, of course, that murderers cannot achieve their own death by murder. It has been suggested that respect for life might be measured by the suicide–homicide ratio. In England, about one-quarter to one-third of murderers commit suicide at the time of the crime. In Denmark the figure is well above 40 per cent. In the U.S.A., on the other hand, suicide-murder is quite uncommon.

Taiwan

In Chinese culture, as it has evolved in Taiwan, delinquency is affected not so much by the immigrant people as by the importation of foreign ideas and customs from the West (i.e. the United States). Formerly, as we have seen, there was no separate youth culture, no traditional framework in which adolescents had a clear sense of their role other than as children or adults. With the advent of Western ideas about the importance of individual liberty and of Western economic influences, a marked change is taking place. These new ideas have made a real impact on the *general* culture. Increasing numbers of youth groups are adopting these ideas, and although adult society is slow to accept them, there is little doubt that the impact of this trend will gain in force until it influences, and eventually transforms, the entire culture.

It is interesting that, in the field of delinquency in Taiwan, two fairly distinct types of young offender can be recognized – the Liu-mang and the Tai-pau (both tending to form groups), who, respectively, represent the traditionalists and the modernists ('Trads' and 'Mods'), and follow either 'Eastern'- or 'Western'-oriented patterns of behaviour (Lin, 1958).

The Liu-mang (or traditionalists) come from the lower classes and are related to the ancient half-tolerated beggar-thieves who hang around the environs of temples. They wear Eastern-type clothing and form rather large groups with a high level of group discipline. They are uneducated, do not include girls in their group, and tend to pursue these youthful group activities until a comparatively late age (20 or over). They may be involved in all sorts of crime, including violence and drug-peddling, and may evolve into more sophisticated adult offenders.

The Tai-pau, on the other hand, look to the West for many models. They wear Western clothes (highly coloured shirts and jeans), are better educated, of middle-class origin, sometimes include girls in the group, tend to be younger (14–18), often confine their delinquency to simple theft or adventurous crime such as car or bicycle stealing, do not take drugs, and operate in relatively small groups. They sometimes become involved in fights with the Liu-mang; if so, they usually lose and either disperse or join the Liu-mang.

132

The Tai-pau represent an essentially middle-class type of rebellious delinquency – of the sort which in England is called 'proving' – and the outlook is similar, that they will grow out of this activity in a year or two unless they are driven into closer collaboration with more serious delinquents by injudicious punishment.

In any case, throughout the East – in Ceylon, Thailand, Pakistan, and the Philippines, there are similar groups of 'Western'-oriented youths in a state of rebellion against traditionalist parents. Education and economic conditions are on their side; when they go to school, they learn to speak a better type of dialect than their parents and are likely to get the better type of commercial jobs since, unlike their fathers, they can speak some English. This trend is also reinforced by the influence of the mass-media, which, as elsewhere, essentially reproduce the 'Western' stereotypes.

Although much is written in the West about the possibility of an increase in middle-class delinquency, it seems probable that it is a more noticeable feature of delinquency in Eastern countries, as well, perhaps, as in the U.S.S.R.

United Kingdom

The United Kingdom comprises a single culture, with Scottish and Welsh culture 'variants' of considerable complexity. Whether Eire forms a separate culture or a 'variant' is not clear. The island position has led to considerable homogeneity, with a socially stratified society which foreign observers regard as more 'feudal' than the inhabitants do themselves. Since the Industrial Revolution occurred very early, and since there has never been much land available for large estates, the ruling class has perhaps been for nearly a century a delicate mixture of aristocracy and plutocracy. Changes have been more gradual than in some countries. The monarchy has been able to encourage standards of integrity and respectability in the leadership, though critics would say that this also encourages the national vice of hypocrisy. There has at least been little indication of organized crime or large-scale illegal exploitation. The success of moderate radical political movements, and the long tradition of unpaid activity in local government, have preserved a *variety* of opportunities for achievement, and many different types of high status. One may still be poor, powerful, or respected, though some would say that this is changing and that an 'achievement' society is developing with wealth as the only accepted form of success.

Two world wars have not, as in some countries, led to the devaluation or discredit of the ruling class, but have produced large economic and social changes, with progress in construction of a 'welfare state' and more equal educational opportunities for all.

In spite of these changes, there has been a disappointingly steady increase in juvenile crime, especially marked in the last five to ten years, during which period the almost universal post-war increase in delinquency has been subsiding in some other European countries. One must remember, however, that, as Sellin (1951) has said, '. . . generally speaking, all criminal statistics are, in fact, statistics of law-enforcement in the broad sense of that term'. The Topeka Conference made it clear that the image of the British in the eyes of foreigners is one of punishing crime with speed and severity. There seems no doubt that the speed of justice is much greater than in most countries; perhaps speed gives the impression of severity, as indeed some judges seem to hope.

In England and Wales crime rose sharply (by one-half) in the Second World War. After the war there was an increase until 1951, followed by a steady decline so that there was not much difference between the levels in 1951 and 1957. Since 1957 there has been a renewed increase, especially in the last few years. Crimes of violence and sex crime, though still constituting only a small proportion of total crime, have increased every year. The most novel feature, however, has been the sharp rise in crime in the age group 16–21, which increased threefold since 1938 and resulted, among other changes, in an increase in the borstal population from 2,800 in 1956 to over 4,400 in 1958, an increase of 57 per cent. Between 1958 and 1962 indictable offences recorded by the police again rose by 43 per cent. One-third of all those found guilty of indictable offences each year are under seventeen, and one-half are under twenty-one. Two-thirds of those found guilty of breaking and entering offences are under twenty-one. Some part of the increase in crimes reported is probably due to the strengthening of police forces (by 9 per cent), readier reporting to the police, and better recording by the police. But, even so, the actual volume of crime has increased substantially.

Indictable offences by juveniles have increased from 0·9 per cent of the relevant age group in 1938 to 1·8 per cent in 1962 among boys; among girls, they have proportionately increased much more – from 0·06 per cent to 0·2 per cent in these years, though still, of course, at a very low level. Towards the end of the Second World War there was a sharp increase in the birth rate, with its peak in 1947; this is commonly referred to as 'the bulge' in the population. Wilkins (1960) has made an analysis of the crime-proneness of the different age groups. The 'bulge' itself has so far been less delinquent than average – in 1955 when there were many more eight-year-olds than before, their crime rate was at its lowest: it was highest in 1948 when they were much fewer. The principle conclusion, however, was that the groups of children born during the period 1935/6–1941/2 had a crime rate above average for all ages from eight to twenty, and were in fact a delinquent generation: and this applied to girls, as well as to the population of Scotland, where crime was recorded differently. These children were, of course, aged four or five during the period of the 1939–45 war. 'It seems that disturbances of social or family life had the most marked effect on subsequent criminality if they occurred when the children concerned were passing through their fifth year' (Wilkins, 1960). There are many possible explanations of this phenomenon; for example, that it is when social relations with contemporaries outside the home are being formed that distorted social patterns are most likely to be learnt.

An exception to this rule is provided by the recent wave of crime in those who were 17–21 in 1960. 'It seems that this pattern is an example of a wave of a different type from those seen earlier in this birth group, for other birth groups and for females. This seems to indicate that the recent crime-wave phenomenon among young males cannot be dismissed as "only to be expected in view of their childhood experiences". Some increase in criminality might have been expected, but not to the extent found to occur' (Wilkins, 1960).

The existence of a delinquent generation of this kind has been questioned by Prys Williams (1963), who suggested that the effect was removed if non-indictable offences were taken into account. Walters (1963) has also suggested that a false impression of a delinquent generation might be created by the marked decrease in delinquency in young children (possibly due to a change in police practice) and the 'crime wave', at the same time, of the 17–21 group.

Crimes of violence have increased considerably, though the

proportion is very low – 2 per cent of all indictable offences. Between 1950 and 1960 they increased by 152 per cent, from 14 to 34 per 100,000. Of these more serious assaults, nearly all consisting of felonies or malicious woundings, almost one-half are street fights or brawls near bars, cafés, etc. and one-third are domestic fights with wives, neighbours, or workmates. The use of weapons is rare; only 10 per cent of assailants had any blunt or sharp instrument with them from the beginning of the fight. The use of firearms is very uncommon – a fact which no doubt explains the public alarm if there are three or four shootings in London a week.

In the present context, this increase has many interesting features. From their detailed investigation of violent crimes in London in 1950, 1957, and 1960, McClintock et al. (1963) concluded that, '. . . although it is generally agreed that in the last ten years there has been an increase in crimes of violence . . . it would be erroneous to assume that most, or even a large part, of the *recorded* increase is due to an actual increase in violent behaviour'. Several factors are involved. (1) A purely administrative change in the reporting by the police of crimes of violence; together with a 'cultural' change in police attitude to reporting of aggressive offences – (e.g. a senior police officer remembered that many years before, as a constable, he had arrested a burglar who fought with him and cut his lip, but was finally overpowered. The station sergeant had said, 'You can't expect burglars to be gentlemen. Brush your coat, wash your face, have a cup of tea, and get back on the beat.' Nowadays, the burglar would be charged with an indictable offence of assault (either causing actual bodily harm or resisting arrest). (2) There is a greater readiness on the part of the public to report offences of violence. As a policeman said '. . . it is a pity that today so much police time is taken up in dealing with public-house brawls or domestic difficulties when it is a foregone conclusion to all concerned the case will be withdrawn or dismissed, or result in binding over the parties to keep the peace. Such incidents were rarely brought to court ten years ago.' Moreover, in slum conditions domestic disputes are common, and there is a tradition of not reporting anything to the police; in the new housing estates to which families are rehoused, it is no longer 'respectable' to tolerate such violence, or the neighbours refuse to do so. (3) Victims now report assaults more readily, partly for insurance purposes and partly because they are no longer

136

accepted behaviour. (4) Coloured immigrants in certain areas show violence towards one another and sometimes use weapons, which results in serious injury. (5) There are more Irish immigrants in some areas who tend to be 'very aggressive when drunk'. (6) Groups of adolescents 'who are against everybody and everything resort to violence at the slightest disagreement or after a mild rebuke'. Though not a serious problem, they attract attention on new housing estates where this sort of behaviour is surprising, or, with the greater ease of communications today, they visit areas where their behaviour causes alarm.

Although two-thirds of those convicted of indictable aggressive offences are over 21 (and a large proportion over 30), the proportion of those under 21 rose from one-quarter in 1950 to one-third in 1960. The sharpest increase has been in boys of 14–17 (a threefold increase in ten years), but the age group of 17–21 contributes the largest proportion.

An apparent increase in 'hooliganism' by teenagers has caused some concern. It is difficult to investigate this because hooliganism has no very certain meaning; but four sorts of behaviour were considered by McClintock as coming within this vague category: quite unprovoked attacks (usually on one boy by a group of youths); attacks on strangers with very little provocation; attacks on members of the public who tried to control rowdy behaviour; and pitched battle between gangs of youths. About one-third of boys under twenty-one convicted of indictable violence fell into this group, which had doubled in the period from 1956 to 1957.

It is the non-indictable forms of hooliganism, however, which have caused most concern. Damage to property, breaking street lamps, and slashing the seats and breaking the windows of railway coaches are a relatively new phenomenon; it has reached such proportions that some train services have been suspended (Wharton, 1964). Similar activities have been described in the United States (Martin, 1961) and in many parts of the world (Gibbens, 1961; Middendorf, 1960).

A second novelty has been the occurrence of 'teenager riots' in which scores of teenagers congregate and generally disturb public order. Those occurring in England in 1964 bear a striking resemblance to those which occurred throughout Germany as long ago as 1956–8, suggesting a surprisingly traditional element of conventionality in this behaviour. The riots occur spontaneously, or as a result of some entertainment (characteristically, the musical film *Rock around the Clock*), or as a 'return' riot a week after the previous one. Those taking part, as in Copenhagen and Germany, are not known delinquents and usually come from every social class. The origins are certainly obscure and are part of 'teenage culture'. A recent complication is the interesting division, among teenagers themselves, into 'Mods' and 'Rockers', who have occasionally come into conflict with one another. They are divided mainly by clothing and dance fashions but, in general, the Rockers are strongly 'masculine' in orientation, wearing leather clothing and driving fast motorbikes, and prone to adopt aggressive attitudes (as do also their girl-friends), while the 'Mods' wear more decorative, exotic, and sometimes effeminate fashions, and adopt a cynical rather than an aggressive attitude to adults. These groups are not necessarily connected in any way with defiant behaviour of an indictable kind, though the public commonly believe that they are.

It is suggested that modern industrialized societies take little notice of the needs of the young and expect adult behaviour from them too persistently. Older cultures provide festivals, carnivals, and other traditional public holidays when orgiastic behaviour is accepted and ritualized. Very similar 'rags' by university students have long been received with indulgence rather than alarm.

Since the Second World War especially, England has been presented with a number of immigration problems of great cultural interest and relevance to the issue of culture conflict and crime. Apart from the Polish emigré forces who settled well in agricultural work after the war (and have preserved many features of Polish culture), and a small number of Hungarians after the rising, the main groups have been Irish, coloured workers from the Commonwealth and Colonies (mainly West Indians and Pakistanis), and immigrants from Cyprus and Malta. There are several other immigrant groups, such as Italian agricultural workers.

The total number of these immigrants is not certain, but they have several features in common. Those who come to England do so because there are much better opportunities than at home of earning a living. In general, they are young adult males, able and willing to work hard and often for longer hours than the English; and they are either single or, if married, come without their wives and families, at least in the early years. There has not been time for the West Indians and Pakistanis to produce a second generation but there are, of course, many generations of Irish in England. In other respects these immigrants are, of course, very different.

Irish (about 2 per cent of the population) and Commonwealth or colonial immigrants (mostly coloured) have contributed a good deal to the increase in indictable crimes of violence between 1950 and 1960. In 1950 the two groups together were responsible for 16 per cent of convictions in London and in 1960, 25 per cent – a much higher proportion than their density in the population. While the English proportion of these offences rose by 80 per cent, the Irish proportion rose by 152 per cent and the coloured proportion by 320 per cent; this is almost entirely limited to adults (McClintock & Gibson, 1961).

Generally speaking, there is little spontaneous colour discrimination in England, but local tension has occurred at times, largely due to competition for housing. Unscrupulous white landlords have exploited the immigrants' willingness to pay high rents while living in overcrowded conditions, and have deliberately made use of this situation (and incidentally encouraged latent racial prejudices) to persuade white tenants to leave rent-restricted accommodation so that higher rents may be imposed on the immigrants who will take their place. The background of the West Indians varies widely; some who come from peasant communities have had a strict Christian upbringing and are startled to find the motherland so irreligious (Métraux & Abel, 1957). Others from the cities are more sophisticated (cf. Patterson, 1963). Of the immigrants (Irish and coloured) convicted of violence 40 per cent have previous convictions and, of these, nearly one-half have a previous conviction for violence. West Indians are especially liable to be convicted of domestic violence; in this group, they were responsible in 1960 for 23 per cent of the convictions. Their excitability and the use of weapons turn a moderate domestic quarrel into an indictable offence.

Apart from violence, they are not perhaps involved in crime. In the West Indies, England is regarded as a country which punishes dishonesty severely. The immigrants intend to make their home in England and are anxious to show that they have adopted English standards. Among 500 women convicted of shoplifting, for example, including a court area which had a population of 25,000

West Indians, only one was a West Indian (Gibbens & Prince, 1962).

Being single, or leaving their wives and families at home often for years on end, exposes them to sexual difficulties. Between 1952 and 1962 new cases of venereal disease rose from 13 to 21 per 10,000 persons. In 1962, among male cases treated in 78 clinics throughout England, Wales, and Scotland 44 per cent were born in the United Kingdom, 28 per cent were West Indians, and 27 per cent other immigrants: 12 per cent of female cases were West Indian and 10 per cent other immigrants. The problem varies widely with locality; nearly 90 per cent of West Indians were treated in London or in four other large cities. They do not, however, tend to be convicted of violent sex offences; in London, only 3 per cent of these offenders were from the Commonwealth or colonies (cf. Brit. Med. Assoc., 1964; Watt, 1961).

The Irish, so close, in the Englishman's eyes, in affection and loyalty, yet with such marked and unique cultural differences, give rise to the most interesting form of culture conflict in England. The full details cannot be discussed here, but are developed in a symposium by a group of distinguished Irish writers (O'Brien, 1954). The Dubliner, Professor Mathew Russell (1964), has discussed the Irish delinquent in England. In 1961, the Irish-born constituted 2 per cent of the population in England and Wales, and in 1951 also formed 2 per cent of the population of Greater London. In 1961, 8 per cent of the male prison population and 9 per cent of the female prison population were Irish-born. We have seen that from 1950 to 1957 the proportion of those convicted of indictable crimes of violence who were Irish rose from 10 per cent to 14·6 per cent; nearly half of these men had been in England for more than five years. In relation to robbery in London (McClintock & Gibson, 1961), 7 per cent of those convicted in 1950 were Irish, and no less than 20 per cent in 1957. The comparison with 2 per cent of the population, however, is not quite fair, for most Irish are probably young single men. If they were all in this category, indeed they would constitute 12 per cent of the single male population of London aged between fifteen and forty. The proportion of 20 per cent of convicted robbers in 1957, however, is distinctly high.

Irish girls are often regarded as liable to take very readily to prostitution in England but, as Russell (1964) shows, 14 out of 140 first arrested for prostitution in London in 1961 were Irish, 5 out of 56 in Brighton, 14 out of 136 in Manchester.

As Russell says, the average Irishman who gets into trouble is the unmarried labourer. 'The single man has two main occupations: work and drink. He has no family in England, few hobbies, few friends and is unwilling to join clubs or organizations of any sort. In Birmingham, where there is a large contingent of young Irish people, the number who join the Catholic Youth Clubs is negligible; in Cardiff, the Irish organizations, formerly flourishing, are now defunct. One of the main characteristics of the Irish emigré is that he is completely absorbed in any culture he joins and nowhere in the world forms an Irish community (with the possible exception of the police in New York!)' (O'Brien, 1954). He works very hard, lives as cheaply as possible in poor lodgings, sends some money home (only an average of £7 a year), and spends most of the remainder on drink. When drunk, he is apt to commit offences of violence. Often, like other immigrants, he gives the impression of such fear of poverty that material security is the only object in life: whether married or not, a sex-life or family life is a luxury that one can easily dispense with. Among 270 clients of prostitutes interviewed in a V.D. clinic (Gibbens & Silberman, 1960), 10 per cent were Irish labourers. They were sharply distinguished by being quite solitary but hard-working, being very heavy drinkers, unwilling to go with prostitutes but being picked up by them (and often robbed) when drunk: these incidents were usually referred to as a great waste of money, and one man even asked if he could be castrated.

The Irish delinquent in England is especially interesting because of the unusual relation of internal and external controls.

At home, the Irish population is one of the few which has steadily declined for over a century from $6\frac{1}{2}$ millions in 1841 to $2\frac{1}{4}$ millions today. For this, there are three reasons. 'For more than a century, Ireland has had the highest emigration rate in the world, the lowest marriage rate in the world, and the latest marriage rate in the world' (O'Brien, 1954): 73 per cent of males and 59 per cent of females between 15 and 44 are single, as contrasted with 30 per cent of American men and women. The average age of marriage in 1946 was 35 for men and 29 for women. If emigration stopped, the nation would increase, and it would also do so in spite of emigration if people married as in other countries. In recent years there has been some increase. The non-marrying habit even persists among the Irish in America (O'Brien, 1954): in the 160 years in which sixty thousand French in Canada have become three and a half million, five million Irish in America have become seven million.

What emerges from the description of Father O'Brien and his colleagues is a complexity of economic and emotional factors profoundly affecting a certain pattern of external and internal controls not found in the English. The rural Irish remain unmarried, waiting to inherit a farm from their parents but not marrying even when economically able to do so, perhaps because of maternal over-protectiveness and dominance (Jones, E., 1923). At the same time, a powerful church maintains a great deal of external social control as well as implanting deep inner controls by putting more stress upon the sinfulness of sex than upon the morality of marriage. The land is poorly developed, and life is whiled away in drinking, horse-racing, and other bachelor activities. Marriage is mainly an economic partnership.

The Irish delinquent youth in England certainly shows clinically the removal of these powerful external controls. He breaks all connections with the church, and does not give his church in England the same status. He thinks of English girls as promiscuous and, after a period of anxious inhibition, becomes more promiscuous than the English. He misjudges the prosperity he sees, is always imagining he could be earning more money even when he is in a good job, and may throw up the latter in pursuit of imaginary improvement.

Where a culture gives rise to the expectation of strong external controls as well as imposing strong internal controls, then the removal of external controls will produce deviant behaviour. But the deviant behaviour is accompanied by much inner guilt, which may increase conflict-ridden deviant behaviour. Guilt may be partly responsible for the heavy drinking and there can be no doubt of the frequency of sexual guilt in the Irish, which in turn is commonly found in certain types of aggressiveness.

U.S.A.

In the United States, the cultural determinants which have led to an exceptionally high level of delinquency as well as material prosperity have to be sought in history. Until 1840, immigrants were mainly English-speaking. Thereafter, many nations supplied immigrants whose number was quite uncontrolled before 1880 and only seriously limited in quite recent times. Between 1900 and 1907 there was a large influx from Southern and Central Europe. Slave labour added a further complication, and later immigration included East Indians, Chinese, and Japanese. The conquest of the West of North America, in the pioneering, 'frontier period' of expansion, not only involved the quest for wealth, and provided considerable opportunities for speculation and gain, but at the same time led to widespread political corruption, as well as unscrupulous and dishonest practices on the part of many 'settlers', in the new territories. Books such as *Our Business Civilization* (Adams, J. T., 1929) describe widespread corruption in the political life of large cities. Later, at the turn of the century, the power of political bosses and machines decreased under the growth of welfare services which replaced the benefits they had manipulated. Codes of ethics, however, are still frequently discussed and drawn up by different organizations, suggesting that improvements are still needed.

The arrival of dissident sects, such as the Menonites, some of which had socially divergent norms and came into conflict with the law on such matters as school attendance and army service, may have contributed to the expectation of a certain amount of deviance. Nowadays, the Black Muslims, while insisting upon the strictest moral standards in their members, have some long-term aims that are antisocial (*Life*, 1963; Lincoln, 1964). The United States have always been exceptionally tolerant of non-conforming groups, and some of these have been more successful than others in preserving their own social organization and controls. But this tolerance may have led to special emphasis upon the factor of individual freedom. The cultural attitude to the law, because of this social tradition, emphasizes that it should control other people but not interfere with oneself; in contrast to the traditional European conception of the law by the common man as a protection against the whims of aristocrats or feudal rulers and therefore as the essential guarantee of freedom.

The existence of heterogeneous norms of behaviour which are frequently in conflict must inevitably influence delinquency. The pressure of minority groups and the lack of a general consensus may have produced the phenomenon of hastily passed legislation which sometimes cannot be enforced, and which can be exploited by

143

criminal groups. It is important, in this connection, here to refer to Prohibition, and certain concomitant social factors which, in the United States, have contributed very largely to the development, entrenchment, and remarkable expansion of the serious and widespread phenomena of racketeering and *organized crime* (Barnes & Teeters, 1943; Bell, 1953; Bergen, 1940; Sellin, 1963; Taft, 1942; Tyler, 1962a, b; 1963; Woetzel, 1963).

The American experiment in Prohibition, which lasted from 1920 (when the Eighteenth Amendment – Volstead Act – took effect) until the repeal of this law at the end of 1933, was, of course, aimed at reducing drunkenness and combating alcoholism. In fact, deaths from alcoholism were at their lowest in 1920, and became, in the next five years, nearly four times as frequent. As Taft (1942) has commented, 'So great was the desire for illicit liquor, that profits from its transportation built up a huge fund to combat the government in its efforts to enforce the law.'

It is not clear what sort of cultural setting permits the development of organized crime. It was found in London in the eighteenth century, and in France during the 'tax-farmer' period of Louis XV; in the Far East today, secret societies are said to flourish as strongly as ever, and the Sicilian Mafia has widely infiltrated the American scene (Allen, 1962). Anthropologists maintain that Americans are great 'joiners of organizations' (perhaps because heterogeneity is uncomfortable), and that criminal behaviour may follow the same rule.

American sociologists, as we have seen, stress the importance in the present situation of the 'delinquent opportunities' created by organized crime in certain cities. When the economic situation leads to prolonged unemployment in the adolescent period, combined with a popular belief that opportunities for great wealth are available to all, delinquent behaviour may seem to offer the only hope of success. Mobility up and down the social scale is rapid, and there is social pressure to display the symbols of financial success. The sociologists also suggest that a high level of violence is tolerated. (When a certain film was made, it was censored in the U.S.A. for its *sex* content. In Sweden, it was censored for its *violence* content, which was not, however, considered exceptional or objectionable in the U.S.A.)

The social and cultural consequences of immigration have been

144

intensively studied in the United States: many of the results have been reported in previous chapters, but many other aspects remain to be discussed (cf. Koenig, 1961).

The U.S.A. is a very large aggregation of population with very varied patterns of behaviour in different areas. One of the conclusions forced upon us when we tried to obtain international information on subcultures is that federations, whether in the U.S.A., Yugoslavia, the U.S.S.R., or other nations, have a cultural bias to discount internal variations. It is not without significance that the home of criminological sociology was Chicago, which offered unusual conditions that may not necessarily apply to more than a few other big cities with similar problems. Alexander (Alexander & Staub, 1939) in fact did not believe that persistent offenders were ever other than neurotic characters, until he emigrated from Germany to Chicago and came to the conclusion that there were psychologically normal persistent offenders. It is all the more to the credit of these authors that they have not been afraid to study these cultural variations.

Many of the influences which affect immigrant behaviour were discussed by Klineberg (1940). 'In the Wickersham report (1933) on Crime in New York State in 1930, it was noted that Mexicans were convicted in great numbers of the crime of carrying concealed weapons; it is obvious that the habits of many Mexicans in their own country have merely been transferred to this one. Beynon's (1934) study of Hungarian peasants in Detroit illustrates a similar mechanism. The Hungarian peasants have transferred to coal stealing from the railroad their old attitude towards the stealing of fire-wood from a nobleman's estate. Groups of boys who steal coal receive, therefore, a sort of social approval in the community, even though this form of behaviour may get them into trouble with the authorities. With the passage of time and the consequent acceptance of American *mores* there is a change in the social patterning of crime. Stofflet (1935) has indicated that the American-born sons of Italian parents commit homicide less frequently than do their fathers, and for different reasons. Whereas in the immigrant group homicide often results from family quarrels and from threats to the family honour, in the next generation it is more likely to be a concomitant of predatory crimes like robbery or burglary.'

According to Lander (1954), many of the foreign-born groups in Baltimore, in 1940, were well integrated culturally and economically

145

in the general community, and were characterized by a high degree of social stability. In at least two of these ethnic groups, the Jews and the Chinese, there was 'almost a complete absence of any recorded delinquency'. Referring to the period 1939–42, he observes that '. . . when other factors are held constant, delinquency rates in Baltimore are highest in areas of maximum racial heterogeneity. In areas of total Negro occupancy, the delinquency rate is no higher than in similar areas of total white occupancy. . . . Futhermore, there are many areas in which the Negro delinquency rate is substantially lower than the corresponding white rate. In two tracts with a population of approximately 200 Negro juveniles, there were no recorded cases of delinquency during the study period.'

Bovet (1951) commented on the very low delinquency rate of the Chinese colony of San Francisco, and drew attention to the fact that this Chinese population had hardly altered its traditional, indigenous way of life. He emphasized, in particular, three basic facts: the strong and stable family setting, on a hierarchical basis; the 'extended' type of family structure; and the extremely tolerant and affectionate attitude of Chinese mothers to their babies. Bovet was led to the cautious, but significant, conclusion that 'It would be rash to affirm without further proof, that there is a correlation of cause and effect between the low percentage of juvenile delinquency and the cultural pattern in this Chinese community. It is, however, impossible not to be struck by the fact that, in these communities, conditions prevail which correspond exactly to the theoretical postulates of depth psychology.'

Further, it appears that much of the community behaviour of the Chinese in America is regulated by self-appointed control groups, and that, in Chicago, they have an official court without political authority, which exercises control over members similar to that maintained in their own country (Barnes & Teeters, 1943; Sutherland & Cressey, 1955).*

The very low crime rate among the Japanese in the United States, and their essentially law-abiding nature, has been attributed to their strong family and community ties. With regard to delinquency among Japanese-American boys, it has been shown that wherever

* It should be noted that in their references to traditional and social conditions in China, all the authors quoted were writing quite some years before the establishment of the Chinese communist régime.

they are closely controlled by the racial colony, they get into little trouble (Hayner, 1942; Hayner & Reynolds, 1933).

Lind (1930) similarly noted that in Honolulu the neighbourhood of concentrated Japanese population had no delinquents; while in the neighbourhood where the Japanese were mixed rather indiscriminately with the rest of the population, several children were brought before the court in one year (cf. the findings, already mentioned, of Lander (1954) in Baltimore).

Reckless (1940) also points out that lack of criminal and delinquent behaviour among the Japanese-Americans is, in his opinion, probably due to 'the amount of isolation, preventing participation in and response to the heterogeneous world beyond the racial colony'.

More recently, De Vos and Mizushima (1962) have undertaken a very thorough survey and assessment of the problems of delinquency in native Japanese and Japanese-Americans respectively. The impression of American teachers is that there is still today, and following the Second World War, almost no juvenile delinquency among Japanese-American youth. 'The question must be raised as to why in the United States young people of Japanese ancestry have been almost without delinquency problems, whereas ethnically similar youth in Japan show similar trends to those true for the United States generally.'

As these authors observe, it is apparent that the Japanese who come to the United States 'were a selective component of their own society' – a process to which they refer as 'selective migration'. This ethnic group 'had strong achievement motivation, quite characteristic of the Japanese farming class generally. Moreover, their attitude toward law and community was such that they had a very high respect for government agencies and community sanctions. When they restructured themselves into communities in the United States, they perpetuated their value with respect to the community as a social force, and they formed very stable family units. . . . In every instance where large populations have immigrated to the United States, they came from a selective part of a total culture. Each immigrant group met the challenge of acculturation to American society somewhat differently. . . . In some cases, the community and family structures that would hold individuals in cohesive units in the old countries did not meet the challenge well in the new environment. . . . The problems in groups with high delinquency rates are

L   147

related to such questions as family and community cohesiveness and sanctions.'

With regard to the significance of racial homogeneity and community cohesiveness, Savitz (1962) has also stated: 'It may be that the negative features generally attributed to migration come into play only when the number of migrants in an area is small and/or the creation of some ghetto-like neighbourhood is not permitted the migrant population.'

Eaton and Weil (1955) have emphasized the effectiveness of the Hutterite communities in the United States in maintaining a social system 'relatively free from individuals . . . who engage in severely antisocial acts – against either their own group or the larger American society'. The various sectarian regulations, issued by the leaders over the years, illustrate the persistent efforts of the Hutterites to control rates of social change by defining the areas in which it is to be approved. When the pressure (both from 'outside', and from inside the colonies) becomes too strong, and the rules are violated widely enough to threaten respect for law and order, 'the Hutterite leaders push for formal change of the written law before it makes too many lawbreakers'. The authors state: 'This process of change might be designated as *controlled acculturation*. It is the process by which one culture accepts a practice from another culture, but integrates the new practice into its own existing value system. It does not surrender its autonomy or separate identity, although the change may involve a modification of the degree of autonomy. . . . The process of controlled acculturation cannot be continued indefinitely without ultimately resulting in more assimilation. . . . In time, the changes may accumulate to bring about a major shift in values, which could destroy the group's existence as a separate ethnic entity.'

In discussing the nature and effectiveness of social controls in ethnic minority groups, e.g. in the United States, many sociologists seem curiously enough to have largely failed to appreciate or, indeed, even to consider the importance of *cultural* factors themselves. De Vos and Mizushima (1962) have commented on this point, as follows: 'Although a great deal of research has compared differences among children of various ethnic backgrounds, very little attention has been paid in these studies to any concept of culture or cultural background as related to the observed differences. Indeed, in recent studies there is a tendency to equate class differences with ethnic differences and to attribute to class background factors more properly considered as ethnic-cultural variations. . . . The problem basic to research in the 'twenties and 'thirties was the possible presence of racial differences in intelligence. The problem today has shifted to the possible effects of differential socialization within cultural groups.'

From data such as have been reviewed in the present section, it would in fact appear that, for such ethnic minority groups, there are two possible ways in which a *'law-abiding' community* may be maintained and reinforced in the first place; viz. (i) by the preservation of the original cultural *integrity*, through relative *isolation* of the group and its traditional social and family organization and norms; or (ii) by the process of cultural *transformation*, and progressive *integration* in the predominant socio-cultural medium.

This is not, of course, to deny the undoubted, though relative, importance in the social adjustment and stability of ethnic minority groups, of the several concurrent or consequent factors which are so frequently emphasized: e.g. isolation from, or contact with, delinquent subcultures and activities; and the influence and pressures of unequal and depressed social, educational, and economic status and opportunity (cf., e.g., Johnson, G. B., 1941; Moses, 1947).

Our American participants, however, emphasized regional differences. In agricultural middle-western States, for example, family life has a stronger patriarchal pattern, the father's role being transmitted by obvious example in ploughing, hunting, shooting, and other masculine activities. Delinquency in these circumstances often takes the form of rebellion against too rigid a paternal domination by a boy who, through wider educational opportunities, has learnt to adopt more flexible attitudes. Such a pattern is in sharp contrast to the mother-dominated family life of the big-city dweller, where the father is often away or adopts a role that is quite unclear to the child.

U.S.S.R.

Unfortunately, no one at the Topeka Conference was able to give information about juvenile delinquency in the U.S.S.R. There can be few countries from which such information would be of more interest in relation to cross-cultural differences, the effect of various forms of social control, or, indeed, the definition of varieties of social deviance. In any case, the available literature is certainly meagre, if we leave aside a number of superficial or else highly prejudiced publications. In two recent articles, however, Beermann (1962a,b) has drawn attention to interesting developments. While these mainly concern legislation, they must necessarily reflect the evolution of public attitudes.

It is hardly necessary to stress that the U.S.S.R. is a union of fifteen republics stretching from Europe to the Far East, and comprising a great range of ethnic and cultural groups, each of which must surely react very differently to a unifying ideology. The history and cultural background of the associated countries, such as Poland, Czechoslovakia, Rumania, Bulgaria, and Hungary are also so diverse that each would require separate consideration, though there is some evidence that juvenile delinquency in these countries generally tends to follow patterns which are more closely comparable to those of Western Europe (Sanford, 1963).

As Beermann (1962) observes, the phrase of St Paul – 'if any would not work, neither should he eat' (2 Thessalonians iii.10) – is made explicit in the present (1936) constitution of the U.S.S.R. 'Both the Pauline and Marxian ideologies aimed at a radical democratisation of life with a revaluation of former values. Such changes are bound to create great ambiguities and uncertainties, causing, at least for some people, considerable anxieties. . . . The borders of that sphere circumscribed by the moral order and the law are shifted, and their outlines are by no means so noticeable and visible as they were. Such a situation must leave a number of persons beyond the pale of socially effective or socially approved life. New offences, hitherto unknown, will be committed, or their anxieties may render some persons incapable of participating in work altogether.'

The Criminal Code of 1926 provided that a socially dangerous action, if not mentioned in the Code, was punishable according to that article of the Code whose definitions were nearest to the act committed. These provisions became increasingly unpopular, especially with Russian lawyers and members of the Procuracy. After Stalin's death and the Party Congress of 1956, greater stress was laid on 'socialist legality'. The provision was abolished in the Code of 1961. In the course of those five years, however, new proposals were made – 'an intensification of the fight against anti-social parasitic elements'. The proposal divided idlers into those living at home (persons living on unearned incomes) and those without permanent residence (vagrants). It is interesting that only eight of the Republics passed the new law – mainly those in the Asian sector. In the Western Republics they were subject to some criticism and were only passed in a modified form in 1961. These laws of the Western Republics shifted the emphasis from the beggars, vagrants, and socially inadequate individuals to the more prosperous categories, i.e. the profiteers and persons enjoying a conspicuous consumption without 'known' sources of corresponding income. A large part of food production (e.g. half the potato and vegetable produce and 80 per cent of the eggs) comes from private rural and urban allotments, and although there are legal provisions for marketing produce, there are local and financial incentives to by-pass them. In the Eastern Republics conditions are again quite different, and there have been cases of bribery and large-scale embezzlement and fraud involving state property. The Criminal Code provides sanctions against certain local, ethnic customs such as tribal feud, payment for brides, or abduction of brides. The population in these areas has not long progressed from a patriarchal way of life which Beermann (1962b) believes '. . . is not conducive to the internalisation of norms of conduct. These remain somewhat external and conduct is governed by tradition.' One main emphasis of the law in the U.S.S.R., therefore, is directed against what we would call 'white-collar criminals', and the Ukrainian 'parasite law' explicitly includes persons who 'manifestly live beyond their earned incomes'. At the same time, the law relating to sexual behaviour seems to demand a high moral standard, as did William Penn and the Quakers in Pennsylvania. We referred earlier to the strict control of prostitution and the method of ridiculing the male clients of prostitutes by putting their names on public notice boards. The 'parasite law' does not apply to juveniles (under 18), or to the elderly, or to the infirm.

The Soviet attitude to juvenile delinquency seems to have passed through successive phrases of great cultural interest (Beermann, 1962a). In the nineteen-twenties the age of criminal responsibility was eighteen years in most cases, and according to Beermann the predominant attitude was expressed by Kufayev, who maintained that '. . . every punishment has a maiming influence on the child. . . . If you desire to have healthy successors, children with their own initiative, and not some docile beings, you should never and under no circumstances punish them.' Later, a more authoritarian attitude developed, responsibility was lowered to twelve years for serious offences, and all juveniles were subject to trial by district courts for juveniles. These provisions were abolished in 1938. Criminology lost its right to be considered a serious subject and was dismissed in encyclopedias (1953) as 'a bourgeois science of crime and the criminals'. From 1956, however, many reforms and modifications took place with an emphasis on education and social treatment, culminating in the law on commissions for cases of juveniles (1961) which combined in a very interesting way most aspects of child care and delinquency control. Criminal responsibility now begins at fourteen years, but only for serious crimes; in general, the offender between the ages of sixteen and eighteen is dealt with as a juvenile delinquent.

The Commissions for juveniles, comprising teachers, doctors, youth organizers, ministry officials, and others, are appointed by executive committees of soviets at all levels. Those at district level have only judicial powers, the higher commissions (republic level, etc.) exercise directive powers in relation to planning for the prevention of delinquency and of neglect. The district commissions have three groups of activities – (1) Welfare and employment. They must detect children in need of care or protection, find employment or education for adolescents, see that welfare and working conditions for adolescents are maintained in industry, and advise parents. No person under eighteen years can be dismissed from work or expelled from school without their consent, and they must find them alternative work or education. They inspect schools, remand homes, and residential institutions, and hear complaints from children or staff. (2) They are responsible for the probation and aftercare of children discharged from special educational or 'medico-educational' institutions, they supervise delinquents on probation and provide employment for them, or organize their supervision by parents or work-collectives. (3) They have judicial functions in relation to all children under fourteen years; and for all those between fourteen and eighteen unless the court, prosecutor, or examining magistrate decides to deal with the case. They have power to demand a public or private apology, to admonish, impose a fine, or (for those over eleven years) remove the juvenile to a special educational institution for not more than three years. They have some powers over the parents of delinquents and can fine them or recover the cost of special education. Their decisions are taken on a simple majority vote of the members of the commission present, they can call for written and oral evidence, and must give their decision in writing 'and with reasons given'.

The district commissions appear to combine the powers which are distributed in England between the juvenile courts, the local authority children's department, and a local branch of the Home Office inspectorate; but they seem to have wider positive powers to provide employment and to supervise the conditions of employment and indeed most other aspects of the lives of children under eighteen, i.e. certain 'youth service' functions which are still widely discussed in Western countries.

Recent visitors (Perry & Stone, 1963) have referred to the informality, the benign exercise of authority, and the close relationship between the law and pedagogy which characterized what they saw, as well as the great variety of the group pressures exerted on the individual. Sandford (1963) was 'reminded of the reports of Japanese society . . . where there seemed to be great homogeneity of standards and the highest continuity of family and community life – and very low delinquency rates'. Recent reforms of higher education – the 'work study' programme – were, however, partly justified on the grounds that they would 'discourage hooliganism, stylism and delinquency in the children of rich parents'. The word 'hooligan' in this and other reports probably has a much wider meaning than in the West. It might be expected, in a society where advancement depends very closely on talent and educational progress, that those young people who do not have enough talent, but are brought up in the homes of successful parents in a relatively privileged position, will face relative frustration and confusion of aspirations. This sort of middle-class delinquency is not unknown in the West.

Such hints as are available suggest that the delinquent in the lowest social class is less of a problem in the U.S.S.R. than the white-collar criminal, the racketeer, and possibly the middle-class delinquent. As is well known, in recent years those found guilty of large-scale frauds and rackets (i.e. crimes seriously threatening the national economy) have been subject to the death penalty. Unfortunately, information is inadequate to allow a general comparison which would certainly be of the greatest interest (cf. also Field, 1955; Rogovin, 1961; Roucek, 1961).

West Africa*

In West Africa, juvenile delinquency is almost non-existent as a problem.

In Niamey (Republic of Niger), between 1953 and 1964 there has been an average of eight reported cases of delinquency a year in the capital. In Bamako (Republic of Mali), in the last four years less than ten cases of delinquency a year have been reported. Since 1953, there has been a 'centre de Rééducation' in Bollé (a small village near Bamako) which, however, only has six inmates (the seventeen others who had been sent there in the previous five years have already been placed in employment, mainly in nationalized concerns). Of these twenty-three cases, nine were the result of paternal requests for (official) correction approved by the courts; the remainder were cases of petty theft and pilfering (food from the markets, etc.). Organized gangs do not exist; collective delinquency is attributable to fortuitous and transient groups.

In Ouagadougou (Republic of Upper Volta) the situation was identical. In 1963 Nouakchott (Republic of Mauritania) had no delinquents.

In Dakar (Republic of Sénégal), a town of some 200,000 population, inquiries show that since 1953 less than 1,300 cases of delinquency altogether had been dealt with through official channels – about 160 cases in the first year, with a gradual annual decrease to about 70 in 1962: 90 per cent were boys aged 13–18 years, with a maximum age incidence of 16 for boys and 17 for girls. Most of the delinquents were born and brought up in the city itself; this was more especially noticeable in relation to girls, 56 per cent of whom were from Dakar itself. Thirty-six per cent of the delinquents had no permanent domicile. The type of offence was quite minor; there were only three cases of serious assault or homicide in ten years. As we have seen in an earlier chapter, the girls were relatively more often dealt with for assault and wounding (usually such offences took place near wells and the parents lodged a complaint in the hope of obtaining damages). The number of reported cases of prostitution

* This section refers to the former *French* West African territories. For a report on Nigeria, see pp. 125–7.

154

is very small – this society takes a somewhat tolerant view of loose sexual behaviour. In Dakar, 80 per cent of delinquents are first offenders; the number of offences by small groups has increased (as compared with those committed alone), but they consist of minor offences by boys of about twelve years.

These figures were collected not from official reports but by personal inquiry of the local public administrators concerned, with the exception of the figures for Dakar, Sénégal.

This low incidence in the republics of West Africa obviously deserves close study. It is attributed by most experts to the relatively slow development of urbanization and industrialization. Those experts who are politically and administratively responsible have some reason to fear that the situation will deteriorate when their various plans for development begin to take effect; they are consequently concerned as to whether delinquency and progress must necessarily go hand in hand.

Recodification of the laws, in itself, may lead to a sharp increase, as indicated by the more recent figures for 'vagrancy' in Morocco. As Brongersma (1964) has observed, before Morocco achieved independence and set up (in 1959) its own penal code (founded largely on the French Code), there were four different systems of law – Arab law, Berber law, Jewish law, and the diverse consular laws of the foreign powers. A man sentenced to two years' imprisonment under one law, for example, successfully appealed that he was under the jurisdiction of another, and was consequently fined the equivalent of eight dollars for the same offence.

In many other areas of the world, as is well recognized, a higher incidence of delinquency has almost invariably accompanied the break-up of traditional (tribal and family) ties, and it is, therefore, almost certain that this trend will similarly continue in West Africa. When this fundamental social disruption is combined with changes in the law – which are in process of adaptation to the cultural norms of the peoples concerned – a substantial and progressive increase in delinquency can be expected. One example, already mentioned, of such legal change, is the Moroccan law on vagrancy. In West Africa, however, there has so far never been any question of including this type of behaviour in the list of juvenile offences, because, traditionally, the abandoned or vagrant child simply does not exist in that cultural area. The social structure, on the one hand, provides un-

failingly for any member of the community, young or old; and, no
the other hand, vagrancy is very largely concealed, in its very diverse
manifestations by the phenomenon of African 'mobility', associated
as this is with the homologous traditional hospitality. Some of the institutionalized actions initiated by external powers have been mis-
interpreted and abused. One of the worst, for example, was *la chasse
à l'enfant* ('the child hunt') organized in some urban areas in order to
fill, in their early days, the centres established for juvenile delinquents. On the other hand, there have been high-ranking magistrates
who have been determined to use the norms of the community
within the terms of the law. When, for example, a polygamous
father, incapable of facing a situation resulting from his own neglig-
ence, complains that he cannot control his children, some magistrates
would severely rebuke him and warn him that, if he did not improve
his parental behaviour, he would be liable to arrest and imprisonment.

Experts in the field have become aware of the dangers of rapid
formulation of new laws, and especially the indiscriminate application of European codes. Under the influence of changing social
attitudes and values, and with two systems existing which have not
been harmonized, it is possible for behaviour which is completely
accepted by traditional rules to be illegal under the new penal code.
This situation was, of course, by no means unknown to the earlier
colonial administrations. Thirty years ago Manuel Gamio (1935),
when discussing the penal code of Mexico, observed: 'Our legislators
make laws for the dominant minority, similar in race, tradition and
civilization to the people of Europe. . . . The social majorities,
especially the indigenous peoples, remain outside the boundaries of
these laws which ignore their biological needs and the nature of their
mental processes, their peculiar indo-hispanic cultures, their
economic status, aspirations and tendencies.'

Today, however, the situation tends to be reversed. It is the
socially sophisticated legislators of the more developed countries
who strain themselves not to impose alien standards upon a culturally distinct, and undeveloped, people; while the indigenous legislators of the newly emerging countries are anxious, indeed over-
anxious, to give no respite to the more backward group within their
countries but to expose everyone to a modern law. It was, after all,
the Moroccan government's own choice or hope that 'a criminal law,
developed in the course of centuries within the Christian-humanistic

tradition of Western culture should, with only slight modification and adaptations, prove to be acceptable in its entirety to a country with a twelve-century history of Islamitic tradition'. Brongersma quotes the Dutch Ambassador in Rabat as saying: 'I know of no people so completely weaned from all xenophobia as the Moroccans.' In Brongersma's view certain changes in the new code have in fact 'a great advantage in terms of broad conception' over the French Code pénal, which 'leaves much to be desired according to modern views' (Brongersma, 1964).

In this last observation we see something of the understandable motivation of the new governments which have multiplied in the last decade, and something of the inevitable rather than mistaken conflict between the old and the new in penal codes. In certain cases, however, the understandable desire to be as up-to-date as possible can nevertheless introduce a danger of false priorities in social legislation. As a recent report of the World Federation for Mental Health (1961) maintained: 'At the present time, however, another – potentially dangerous – consequence of improved international communications is seen in the increasing possibility of a too rapid and uncritical acceptance of new procedures by emerging nations.' One common procedure of this sort is to devise complicated methods of treatment for delinquent children before there is any adequate service to provide abandoned children with a substitute home. Morocco, with its new emphasis upon vagrancy, clearly did not repeat this error.

As an instance of the amount of 'cultural interpretation' which may be needed to reveal the significance of apparently antisocial acts, one may cite the special 'prophetic community' on the Ivory Coast, West Africa, at present being studied by Jean Rouch (1963) and other experts. Belief in the extraordinary and threatening powers of witchcraft as the cause of death, failure of crops, etc. is widespread in forest villages in this part of Africa. The security of the village may be considered to be permanently threatened by men and women who, it is believed, are able to cause harm at a distance, and, especially, to 'eat the flesh' of their victim. Hysterical men and women still believe that they are able to kill the soul, the 'double' of people, and having gained possession of it to cut it up, cook it, devour it, and share it with others (Tauxier, 1932). It is not difficult to find reports of innumerable judicial investigations in the past fifty years, containing detailed allegations concerning witchcraft. In the course of these trials, the accused may freely confess to having killed and 'eaten the flesh' of various people whom they have bewitched. By this, they really refer to the 'double' of the person concerned, and nearly all children and young people who die are assumed to have died of unnatural causes (cf. also Field, 1937; Rattray, 1923; Tait, 1963). There are several communities which practise the method of public confession (often drawn up in legal terms) by the members who have come there to be healed. The research workers studying such a community have collected over five hundred public confessions of individuals claiming to have killed a number of people, drunk their blood, eaten their flesh, etc. Those making the confessions, which are genuinely accepted by the other members of the community, themselves probably believe them to be true, but the police and administrators clearly need to know when to recognize them as false.

Research conducted in Tananarive (Madagascar) by the Centre International de l'Enfance has shown that, as has so often been observed elsewhere, the predisposing factors in theft by children may be attributed to migration of the family to an urban area, separation from traditional backgrounds, lack of opportunity for training in skilled work, etc. (Paul-Pont & Belvèze, 1955; Paul-Pont, 1956). But it is *also* recorded that, in certain ethnic groups in Africa, theft (especially of oxen) is regarded as a sign of virility when committed outside the tribal group, and as a crime only when committed within the tribe. The limits of these traditions are ill-defined and probably not fully recognized by courts of law (Paul-Pont, 1956). – (Cf. also works marked † in Bibliography).

West Germany

Since the Second World War, West Germany has undergone very rapid economic development, comparable with that of Japan. Urbanization and industrialization have been well developed for many years, but have greatly extended; and culturally the society has become what may be called an acquisitive or achieving society. In former times, German society was led by the Prussian agricultural and military *élite* who even influenced the rising economic leadership. The Nazis, however, removed the traditional *élite* from the scene, and since the Second World War business leaders have taken the place of the Prussian State *élite*. German culture tends to rely upon decisions from above – in church, education, or politics; and an achievement orientation has tended to inherit the authority of the older type of leader.

The modern youth culture has made its own spontaneous adjustment to the situation. The old '*Jugendbewegung*' was romantic, naturalistic, with a 'back to nature' orientation (Becker, 1946; Borinski & Milch, 1945), but the present orientation is typical of an industrial urban society and has been a spontaneous development. In the teenage riots of 1956–8, middle-class youths were over-represented compared with the lower class (Bondy *et al.*, 1957). The attempt to evade the rigid middle-class control of their parents causes tension and revolt, which show themselves in very ill-defined rebellious groups. Vandalism is one indication of this kind of revolt. Where the values of the adult society are increasingly based upon financial success, as some American studies have suggested, this may lead to frustration of a new kind in young people who are unable to realize ambitions in this field.

In Germany, there has been a moderate general increase in the rate of convictions, but this is mainly due to a considerable increase in the adolescent age group (18–21), and also, although to a lesser extent, to an increase in convictions of juveniles (14–18). The adult ratio has remained at a fairly steady level, but in children under fourteen there has been an increase. Since adult rates have not increased appreciably during the last ten years, in spite of constant recruitment of the adolescents who were previously so delinquent, one may perhaps conclude that this adolescent behaviour need not be taken too seriously because the majority clearly recover from this phase as they become adult. This improvement after twenty-one is not generally considered to be due to the effectiveness of treatment.

The character of youthful crime has also shown interesting changes. Petty larceny is, as usual, by far the commonest offence, but violent offences and fraud have increased proportionately. Sexual offences by adolescents and juveniles (14–18) have also increased: this age group commits about 30 per cent of rapes, compared with 20 per cent some years ago. The proportion of illegal abortions among girls under twenty-one has risen from 7 per cent to 11 per cent, and cases of infanticide by girls of this age have increased from 21 per cent to 38 per cent. Although arson is not common, a surprisingly large number of such offences are committed by children under fourteen.

Western Germany, also, has had problems of migration. Nearly one-quarter of the present population were not born in the Federal Republic. The available data suggest that the refugee population from what is now Poland have been rather less delinquent than the average, whereas the German refugees from Eastern Germany are slightly more delinquent. The former group have tended to preserve their culture, have arrived in organized units (families, communities), and obtained much financial and other help to enable them to integrate. Those who came from Eastern Germany often came alone, were attracted for a variety of reasons to the new environment rather than expelled from the old, and have in many cases had to 'sink or swim'.*

* It has not been possible here to consider in any detail the important problems of Southern and South-East Asian countries. A few relevant references, among many, may, however, be mentioned: Manshardt, 1959; Ministry of Education, 1954; Murphy, 1963; Sethna, 1952; Unesco, 1956c.

devaluation of the parental image, authority, and influence on the part of children and adolescents, so that it becomes difficult for the latter to internalize the culturally requisite norms of mature adult behaviour.

Yet prolonged segregation of a minority group, whether imposed by the receiving community, or self-imposed in isolated communities, will inevitably lead to an exaggerated awareness on the part of the larger society of the features which distinguish the subculture, and entail the risk of future discrimination and persecution if at any time the dominant culture comes to feel insecure and, consequently, looks for a scapegoat. Few have as yet attempted to determine whether there is an optimum speed of acculturation, dependent perhaps upon such factors as the span of generations, in a given socio-cultural context. There are, however, so many variables involved in every specific instance of this process (and many of them may be unpredictable), that it does not seem very likely that such an assessment could be made with any degree of accuracy. In Israel, attempts to bring about active cultural integration, by scattering immigrants among the established population in the hope of speeding up the assimilative process, proved unsuccessful and resulted in widespread social maladjustment among those concerned. This experiment was, therefore, abandoned in favour of a return to gradual integration, with the preservation of the cultural homogeneity of immigrant groups, and a high level of social adjustment was thus successfully attained. Since a great many countries throughout the world are faced with these problems, it is possible that systematic international comparative studies of social situations before and after immigration might nevertheless help to throw some light on the question of optimum speeds of integration.

Investigations in various schools have shown that the process of learning may be greatly accelerated, where there are educationally constructive groups. It would be of considerable value if a cross-cultural study were made of the groups which tend to facilitate positive or negative learning.

Psychiatrists and also practising lawyers are aware of the potential importance of the many experiments being undertaken at present to determine the most effective forms of treatment. In view of the essentially conservative structure of existing penal systems, it will probably be more useful, primarily, to concentrate on studying the

M   163

problem of who will, and who will not, respond to those forms of treatment which are at present available, rather than to direct *all* society's resources toward the investigation of new and untried forms of treatment. Research projects of this kind are principally delayed by the absence of any generally acceptable nosology of behaviour disorders. Such objective predictive categories as have so far been suggested are inadequate and are constantly in need of modification. We urgently require generally applicable diagnostic criteria which will provide us with the means to test the effectiveness of different methods of treatment.

Psychiatrist participants naturally emphasized the need for intensive studies of the effectiveness of treatment. In medical research, progress has often been made by establishing reliable criteria for making prognoses and assessing responses to treatment, and then reformulating the principles of differential diagnosis in the light of such data. In the international field, many important experiments, in which delinquents are being dealt with in vastly different ways, are in fact constantly in progress in different countries and cultures, although they are not necessarily intended as such. With the help of international and interprofessional teamwork, and extensive follow-up studies planned on an international scale, these very different experiences and practices might be converted into scientific cross-cultural experiments of the greatest value. We know that, for many nations, the larger the number of psychiatric hospital beds, the smaller the prison population, and vice versa (Penrose, 1949). It is most important to find out who are those who respond to the respective types of social action, and why they respond to one type rather than another.

Finally, there is a need for international research which is both interdisciplinary and multi-dimensional. Ferracuti and Wolfgang (1964) have discussed this question in interesting detail, in a paper entitled 'Clinical versus sociological criminology: separation or integration?' Criminologists are still largely divided into two groups. The sociological criminologists, on one hand, tend to elaborate interesting social theories of crime causation although, as we have seen, less and less attention is paid to the empirical validation of these theoretical concepts, and the practical deductions to be drawn from the latter are not always apparent. Psychiatrists and psychologists, by contrast, are so immersed in the practical and clinical aspects of criminology that they have little time or energy to evaluate their theoretical assumptions and conclusions which are often built upon vague and unsubstantiated concepts.

There is, in fact, a sociology of sociologists and of psychiatrists; like everyone else, they are locked within the pressures of their respective 'subcultures'. These subcultures might be explained on the basis of 'differential association' with colleagues, and non-association with their disciplines, leading to constant reinforcement of theories which are not sufficiently tested. But the theory of differential 'opportunities' may also apply! The academic sociologist is presented with opportunities for advancement which demand that he establish new theories, and the pressure to do this may well lead him to undertake the careful observations, and the collection of material, on which they must be based. The psychiatrist, with opportunities for clinical practice, is tempted to expound his convictions about the effectiveness of treatment without waiting for the results of properly controlled testing. In both fields there is a great shortage of scientific data. It is, however, most unlikely that, unless those of us who, in our respective disciplines, are concerned with the human sciences are able to understand ourselves and the inter-personal forces which influence our actions and judgments, we will be able adequately to understand and treat the 'criminal'.

Chapter IX

CULTURE AND
DELINQUENCY: AN OVERVIEW

by Otto Klineberg

Studies of crime and delinquency have followed many different pathways, and the resulting literature is rich and varied. The present inquiry has focused attention on delinquency as a way of life, as a pattern of attitudes and activities acquired by an individual as a member of a particular segment of a specific society. No claim is being made that this is the only valid, or even necessarily the most important, approach. The argument still continues as to whether genetic factors play any significant role, but no one can deny that many cases of delinquency are related to poverty and overcrowding, to the situation within the family, to psychological mechanisms that reach deep into personality. Explanations in terms of culture can never tell the whole story, since every individual makes his own selection from what the culture offers him, accepting certain aspects, rejecting others. Even in areas of greatest frequency of delinquency, there will be many young people who choose a way of life approved by the wider society rather than by their age-mates in the immediate environment.

The fact remains, however, that cultural factors do exert a very real influence, probably greater than is usually realized. The very definition of criminality is culturally determined, varying from one society to another, and from one period of history to another, both in the nature of the relevant legal codes and in the manner in which such codes are interpreted. Murder in defence of family honour may be condoned or condemned; the wide range of sexual activities is paralleled by an equally wide range of laws and of strictness of enforcement; the taking of someone else's property is not everywhere or always a crime; the same is true for suicide and for alcoholism. As far as juvenile delinquency is concerned, truancy and vagrancy may not even be listed among possible offences in certain countries. It is not surprising that many, if not most, investigators have given up the search for *the* characteristics of *the* criminal or delinquent in view of the wide range of behaviours that are (or are not) included in a criminal category.

There are many other ways in which cultural factors enter. The large discrepancy in recorded delinquency for boys and girls, for example, found in all countries for which statistics are available, can best be explained by the different attitudes of society as to what behaviour is expected or accepted from boys and girls respectively. There are great variations in the frequency of delinquent behaviour in children of different ages, as well as changes in such frequency from time to time, which at least to some extent reflect the influence of peer cultures and cannot wholly be explained by the stage reached in biological development. Delinquency in any community will be influenced also by the patterns of behaviour characteristic of the police, the judges in the juvenile courts, and all the other official personnel with whom the young offenders, actual or potential, come into contact; both initial reactions and recidivism may vary considerably according to whether 'they' are regarded as friends or foes.

As far as adults are concerned, many examples could be given of criminal subcultures. Though varying considerably in their character and in their relationship to the larger society, they all represent (or represented) a way of life accepted by the members, who usually followed faithfully and even rigidly all the rules and regulations. Sometimes they included political and even religious aspects. As examples may be mentioned the 'Assassins' of the Middle East, the Dacoits and Thags (Thugs) of India, the Sect Rouge of Haiti, the Camorra of Naples, and the Mafia of Sicily. The 'subculture of violence' characteristic of certain parts of Colombia was originally political in purpose, but later became more indiscriminate in its nature; it represents a particularly interesting case in the present context because young children were frequently recruited as members. At a less extreme level, a tradition of violence has been more characteristic of the South than the North in the United States, and it has been suggested that this may be one of the factors contributing to the crime rate of Negroes, which is much higher for those born in the South.

Although the direct comparison of national crime rates in *absolute* terms is for many reasons difficult, if not impossible, it is easier to establish *relative* differences in the frequency of the types of crime committed. It seems clear, for example, that there is considerably more suicide and less homicide in Denmark than in other (even other Scandinavian) countries; that crimes of violence among the Irish

167

in the United Kingdom are usually committed under the influence of alcohol; that sexual offences are on the increase in the Federal Republic of Germany; that drunkenness is much more frequent in Helsinki and Oslo than in Copenhagen; that there is a relatively high proportion of white-collar crime in the U.S.S.R. and Israel. Biology and race are of no help in explaining these variations; they appear clearly to be a function of cultural differences in the way in which crimes tend to be committed.

Similar variations occur at the juvenile level, and they require a similar explanation. Teenage gangs represent a serious problem in the United States, but are rare in Italy (except in the south) and practically non-existent in Nigeria; there has been considerable violence and rioting in Sweden but very little in Belgium; the use of drugs was exceptionally widespread in Japan, for a time more so than in any other country. In Taiwan there are two distinct varieties of delinquent group, one closer to older, traditional forms of behaviour, the other more 'modern', Western in outlook; in Israel there are also two varieties, distinguished by class, with middle-class delinquency quite different in character from that found among the children of labourers. Immigrant groups contribute more than their proportional share of delinquency in Israel, but less in Canada or Australia.

There are marked cultural differences in the way in which delinquency is handled when it does occur. The infinitesimal amount of delinquency reported for the Chinese in the United States may indicate less deviant behaviour, but is more probably due to the fact that such behaviour is taken much more seriously by the whole (extended) family, and that measures are introduced within the group itself to redress the wrong and punish the offender. The reported rise in juvenile delinquency in Japan may be due at least in part to increasing tension between the generations since the end of the Second World War, with a consequent reduction in the controls previously exercised by the parents.

Familiar to all students of culture is the phenomenon of borrowing, of diffusion of cultural items and patterns of behaviour from one society to another. This is never a mechanical process, since a selection is always made out of the items offered for export; acceptance or rejection will then be related to prevailing needs, or to the degree of coincidence with what is already known or accepted. In connection with the introduction of the Mafia into the United States, this Sicilian pattern took firm hold probably because it found in the New World a soil propitious for its growth and development. At the same time it is highly probable that other Americans saw in the Mafia a form of behaviour which they could turn to good use; they altered their own conduct in the light of knowledge of these 'new' forms of criminal activity. In the field of juvenile delinquency, borrowing and diffusion are particularly striking in connection with the relations between Puerto Rico and the United States. Delinquent gangs were evidently unknown among young Puerto Ricans until their migration to New York and Chicago; there they acquired the habits of gang behaviour. Recently, there has been considerable reverse migration, with many Puerto Ricans returning to their original homes; they have brought back with them the 'American' gang pattern, with a consequent spectacular increase in juvenile delinquency. The rise in narcotic addiction among young Puerto Ricans has been explained along similar lines. In Belgium also it has been suggested that American influence is responsible for the increase in gang behaviour. Crime and delinquency evidently constitute articles of both import and export!

Special problems arise when two different cultures, each with its own standards of acceptability in behaviour, come into contact. Sometimes the results with regard to criminal acts are clear and even predictable, as when Mexicans are arrested for carrying weapons in New York, or Hungarian immigrants steal coal from the railroad tracks in Detroit because they had been allowed to take wood from the nearby forest in their homeland. Sometimes the relationship is much more complex, and 'culture conflict' operates more indirectly as a cause of delinquent behaviour. Italian parents are much stricter than are Americans about letting their daughters go out with a boy unchaperoned; this means conflict between Italian immigrants to the United States and their American-born daughters, and at least some cases of delinquency have their origin in this situation. Puerto Ricans in this respect resemble Italians, and girls who return to Puerto Rico from the United States are regarded as having become 'loose' in their morals – and sometimes are tempted to live up to the reputation thrust upon them. In parts of Africa the break-up of the traditional patriarchal family due to rapid cultural change may mean loss of respect for authority. Such rapid change usually means some degree of conflict, whether it occurs as the result of actual contact through migration, or as a revolution in folkways due to technological development. This does not always or necessarily lead to delinquency, since immigrant groups, and even their children, may be particularly law-abiding. The fact remains that some cases of crime and delinquency can legitimately be attributed to the phenomenon of culture conflict.

The stress on cultural factors in the aetiology of delinquency makes the assumption that this form of behaviour, like any other, may be *learned*. This concept may be disturbing to those who view learning as necessarily conscious, deliberate, and goal-directed; it may be all of these, but it may also occur incidentally, almost by chance. The learning of delinquency may have either of these two sets of characteristics, or both. Imitation of others is rarely, if ever, a blind process. We imitate because we are motivated in some way to do as others do, because we think we can gain something, either materially or in terms of acceptance or prestige, or because imitation has been a rewarding experience in the past. All these factors may play a part in the learning of delinquency. The fact remains that such learning is usually limited to the patterns of behaviour already present in our social environment.

In the light of this analysis, two major questions emerge. The first refers to motivation, the second to behaviour. The first asks *why* delinquency; the second, *what* it is and how it is learned. The present inquiry has stressed the second, but with full awareness of the importance of the first. Further progress will depend on the deepening and extension of our knowledge of both, and of the manner in which they are interrelated.

NOTES ON PARTICIPANTS

in the International Study Group on
Cultural Factors in Delinquency

KLINEBERG, Professor Otto: *Chairman of the meeting*
Professor of Social Psychology at the Sorbonne (University of Paris).
Late Professor, and first Chairman of the Department of Social
Psychology at Columbia University. Has been very active in the
affairs of the World Federation for Mental Health, Chairman of its
Executive Board, etc., and Chairman of a number of committees.

AHRENFELDT, Dr Robert H.
Psychiatrist. Worked with T. P. Rees at Warlingham Park Hospital,
and at Croydon Child-Guidance Clinic. Became particularly interested in maladjusted and delinquent children and adolescents,
which brought him into contact with the Institute for the Study and
Treatment of Delinquency, London, and with Dr Hermann Mannheim. Was for a time Deputy Assistant Director of Army Psychiatry
at the British War Office. Author of *Psychiatry in the British Army
in the Second World War* – which contained a summary of his own
work on the disposal of delinquents in the Army. Consultant and
Research Associate of the World Federation for Mental Health since
1950. Has collected and summarized material for W.F.M.H.,
W.H.O., and for a number of specialized international and interprofessional meetings in the mental health field.

ASUNI, Dr T.
Medical Superintendent, Aro Hospital, Abeokuta. Associate Lecturer
in Psychiatry, University of Ibadan. Was educated in Lagos,
Nigeria, Trinity College, Dublin University, and the Institute of
Psychiatry (University of London). His M.D. thesis was based on his
research on maladjustment and delinquency in London. Has carried
out investigations into attempted suicide and juvenile delinquency
in Western Nigeria, and participated as a lecturer in the 12th
International Course of Criminology in Israel in 1962.

BEATY, Mr William T.
At present Executive Director of the New York office of the World

Federation for Mental Health. Trained in Public Health and social work at the University of South Carolina and Tulane University, Louisiana, etc. For thirteen years Assistant Executive Director of the New York State Association for Mental Health. Has travelled and observed mental health activities and services in the major centres of Western Europe and the Near East.

CHRISTIANSEN, Dr Jr. Karl Otto
Has held a number of different research and educational appointments. Has taught at Herstedvester; was Social Affairs Officer at U.N. Headquarters; Lecturer in Criminology since 1944, University of Copenhagen. Has written on collaborators in World War II, short-term offenders, and a number of articles on juvenile delinquency aud other aspects of criminology. At present engaged on a study of criminality among twins (in co-operation with others).

FERRACUTI, Dr Franco
Professor of Forensic Medicine, University of Rome. Working at the moment for the U.N. as Director of a criminological project of the University of Puerto Rico Social Science Research Centre. Was a Fulbright Scholar, University of Wisconsin. Since 1952 instructor in Psychodiagnostic Techniques in Criminology, the Law School, University of Rome. Member of the American Psychological and Sociological Associations, the International Society for Criminology, and the International Association of Applied Psychology. Author of sixty papers, and one book on the psychological aspects of criminology.

GIBBENS, Dr T. C. N.
Consultant psychiatrist to the Bethlem Royal and Maudsley Hospitals, Reader in Forensic Psychiatry at the University of London, and psychiatrist to the London Remand Home for girls. Joint Secretary of the International Society of Criminology, and a past President of the British Society of Criminology. Consultant on problems of delinquency to the World Health Organization, for whom he has made surveys. Member of the Royal Commission on the Penal System.

GREENWOOD, Dr Edward G.
Child psychiatrist. Menninger Foundation's consultant to children's

institutions, agencies, and schools. Participated in the World Federation for Mental Health International Conference in 1955 and in 1960 was a representative of the Menninger Foundation to the United Nations' Congress on Prevention of Crime and Treatment of Offenders in London. Recently President of the American Orthopsychiatric Association. Member of the Editorial Board of Excerpta Criminologicia Foundation and a member of the Research Advisory Council of the National Research and Information Centre, National Council on Crime and Delinquency.

HALLEN, Mr Philip

President, Maurice Falk Medical Fund, Pittsburg, Pa. Trained in public health and mental hospital administration. Principal previous work was done in hospital and community planning and administration. At present directing the Fund's support of programmes in public health and social psychiatry.

LIN, Dr Tsung-Yi

Professor and Chairman, Department of Neurology and Psychiatry, National Taiwan University, and Director, Paipei Children's Mental Health Centre. Recently Chairman of the Executive Board, World Federation for Mental Health. Major interest is in changes in adolescent and delinquent behaviour in relation to socio-cultural changes in Asian societies.

MAILLOUX, Father Noel

Has a Ph.D. and a Licentiate in Sacred Theology from the Angelicum in Rome (1938). Served as Chairman of the Department of Psychology at the University of Montreal from 1942 to 1957. Currently, Vice-Dean of the Faculty of Philosophy. Was President of the Canadian Psychological Association (1954–5). In 1959 was the recipient of the first Career Research Award presented by the Canadian Mental Health Association. Chairman of the Canadian Corrections Association, and as such was largely responsible for the organization of the International Congress of Criminology to be held in Montreal in August 1965.

MÉTRAUX, Mrs Rhoda

Cultural anthropologist; trained at Yale and Columbia. Overriding interest is in the ways in which people learn their culture, and, in particular, adapt themselves to change. Much fieldwork in the

Caribbean area. Has worked on French, Chinese, and American cultures. At present finishing a project with Margaret Mead on multisensory aspects of learning cross-culturally related to time and space.

MODLIN, Dr Herbert G.
Director, Law and Psychiatry Division, Menninger Foundation; Associate Clinical Professor of Psychiatry, University of Kansas Medical School; Lecturer in Behavioural Science, University of Kansas Law School; Consultant, Medical Centre for Federal Prisoners, Springfield, Missouri; Consultant, Reception and Diagnostic Centre, Kansas State Prison, Topeka; Vice-Chairman, Section on Legal Aspects of Psychiatry, American Psychiatric Association. Assisting in the development of several ongoing investigative projects in the field of juvenile delinquency, and follow-up studies of boys released from industrial school.

MORRIS, Professor Norval
Professor of Law, University of Chicago. Until recently Director, U.N. Institute for the Prevention of Crime and Treatment of Offenders, Asia and the Far East. A graduate of Melbourne, Adelaide, and London Universities; solicitor and barrister. Has been Professor of the Faculty of Law at Adelaide, and teacher in London, and at Harvard and Utah. Publications include *The Habitual Criminal and Studies in Criminal Law*.

NAGEL, Dr William H.
Professor at Leiden University; lawyer and criminologist. Recently in residence at the Menninger Foundation. Has been active in all international activities in the field of criminology and delinquency.

PIDOUX, Dr Charles
Psychiatrist. Ethnologist, West Africa. Has worked in the Medico-psychological Observation Centre for young delinquents at Clermont-Ferrand; in the Bureau for Juvenile Delinquents in the Ministry of Education in Morocco. Technical Consultant to Unesco and to the Institute of Social Science of the Republic of Mali. Member of the International Society of Criminology and of Ethno-Psychology. Interests: sociology and psychology of the populations in the region of the Niger.

RACINE, Mlle Aimée
Professor at the University of Brussels; social psychology; sociology
of education, juvenile delinquency. The latter her main topic for
years; has published a number of books on the subject either alone,
before the war, or in collaboration since her appointment as Scientific
Director of the Centre d'Etude de la Délinquance Juvenile, created
in 1957 under the auspices of the Belgian Ministry of Justice.

RAMAN, Dr A. C.
Specialist psychiatrist and medical superintendent the Brown
Sequard Hospital, Beau Bassin, Mauritius. Is deeply interested in
social psychiatry, and gives part of his time to study the influence
of cultural factors in mental health. Two of his studies have been
published (a) of the effect of rapid culture change on mental health,
and (b) of the eldest child in various culture groups.

RECKLESS, Professor W. C.
Professor of Sociology, Department of Sociology and Anthropology,
Ohio State University, Columbus, Ohio. Has been very active in
research in delinquency, and particularly in the behaviour of peer
groups. Has published many articles and a number of books.

REES, Dr John R.
Psychiatrist. Honorary President, World Federation for Mental
Health (Director 1949–62). Has been concerned all his professional
life with problems of delinquency and their treatment.

SACK, Dr Fritz
Sociologist, qualified in 1958. Teaching and research assistant of the
Sociological Seminar, University of Cologne, with Dr René Koenig.
His dissertation for Cologne University dealt with problems of
deviant and adjustment structures within the economic sector of
German society. Since 1963 has been editorial secretary of the
Kölner Zeitschrift für Soziologie und Sozialpsychologie. Teaching
courses on criminal deviancy and other topics at Cologne. Publica-
tions include an article 'Abweichendes Verhalten' in Bernsdorf-Bulow,
Handworterbuch der Soziologie 1964 and a work in collaboration with
R. Koenig, Kriminalsoziologie, Frankfurt (forthcoming).

SATTEN, Dr Joseph
Psychiatrist and psycho-analyst. Director, Department of Social

Psychiatry, the Menninger Foundation. He is a consultant to the Medical Centre for Federal Prisoners, Springfield, Missouri; Kansas Reception and Diagnostic Centre, Topeka, Kansas; and State Hospital for the Dangerous Insane, Larned, Kansas, as well as a lecturer in the School of Law of the University of Kansas.

SELLIN, Professor Thorsten
Professor of Sociology, University of Pennsylvania; Editor of the *Annals* of the American Academy of Political and Social Science; President, the International Society of Criminology; formerly Secretary-General, the International Penal and Penitentiary Commission. Author of many papers and books on crime and its socio-cultural aspects.

SHOHAM, Dr Shlomo
Director, Institute of Criminology, Ramat-Gan, Tel-Aviv, Israel. The Institute has a training programme for the various services concerned with prevention and control of crime and treatment of offenders, i.e. police, probation service, prison commission, and military police; it also carries out research in the aetiology of crime and delinquency and the results of treatment. Projects in various stages of implementation are, *inter alia*, middle- and upper-class juvenile delinquency, a follow-up study of inmates of a young-adult prison, crimes of passion, delinquency in the Kibbutz. He has published four books and about forty articles.

TWAIN, Dr David C.
Clinical psychologist, with interest in sociology. Has practised as a psychologist in the U.S. army and Public Health service, and then for four years in the Federal Bureau of Prisons. Three years ago became Consultant to the National Institute of Mental Health in the area of crime and delinquency. Is now Chief of Crime and Delinquency, Section of the National Institute for Mental Health. Has strong interest in research and training as they contribute to the development of programmes in the area of delinquency.

REFERENCES

Note. Items marked * are additional references to the section on Israel (p. 115) and those marked † are additional references to the section on West Africa (p. 154).

ADAMS, J. T. (1929) *Our Business Civilization: Some Aspects of American Culture,* New York.

ADAMS, S. (1961) *Interaction between Individual Interview Therapy and Treatment Amenability in Older Youth Authority Wards,* Calif. Board of Corrections, Sacramento, pp. 27–44.

AGRANAT COMMITTEE (1956) *Juvenile Delinquency in Israel,* Ministry of Justice, Jerusalem, Israel.

AHRENFELDT, R. H. (1958) *Psychiatry in the British Army in the Second World War,* London and New York (p. 211 cited).

ALEXANDER, F. (1942) *Our Age of Unreason: A Study of the Irrational Forces in Social Life,* Philadelphia, pp. 218–20.

ALEXANDER, F., and STAUB, H. (1939) *The Criminal, the Judge and the Public,* London.

ALLEN, E. J. (1962) *Merchants of Menace: The Mafia,* Springfield, Illinois.

ALLPORT, G. W. (1937) *Personality,* New York.

—— (1954) *The Nature of Prejudice,* Cambridge, Mass.

ASUNI, T. (1962) Suicide in Western Nigeria. *Brit. med. J.,* **2,** 1091–7.

—— (1963) Preliminary study of juvenile delinquency in Western Nigeria, *Proc. 12th Int. Course Criminol.,* Jerusalem, Israel, **1,** 186–94.

AUBERT, V. (1956) White-collar crime and social structure, *Amer. J. Sociol.,* **58,** 263–71.

BAILEY, D. S. (1955) *Homosexuality and the Western Christian Tradition,* London, pp. 162–3.

BARKER, G. H., and ADAMS, W. T. (1963) Glue sniffers, *Sociol. social Res.,* **47,** 298–310.

BARNES, H. E. (1927) *The Evolution of Penology in Pennsylvania: A Study in American Social History,* Indianapolis.

BARNES, H. E., and TEETERS, N. K. (1943) *New Horizons in Criminology: The American Crime Problem,* New York. Cf. especially: pp. 22–40, 55–76 (Prohibition and Organized Crime); 41–55 (White-collar Crime); 125–31 (Immigration as a Factor in Criminality); 182–202 (Race and Crime).

BATAWIA, S. (ed.) (1960–4) *Archiwum Kryminologii*, Warsaw, **1**, and **2** [in Polish, with English summary].

BATESON, G., and MEAD, M. (1942) *Balinese Character: A Photographic Analysis* (Special Publ. New York Acad. Sci., Vol. 2), New York.

BAU CARPI, J. L. (1961) Aspects of juvenile delinquency in the world and in Spain, *Rev. Obra Protec. Menores*, **18**, 14–26. Abstract in: *Excerpta criminol.*, 1962, **2**, 180-1.

BECKER, H. (1946) *German Youth: Bond or Free*, London.

BEERMANN, R. (1962a) The Soviet law on commissions for cases of juveniles, *Brit. J. Criminol.*, **2**, 386–91.

—— (1962b) The parasite law in the Soviet Union, *Brit. J. Criminol.*, **3**, 71–80.

BELL, D. (1953) Crime as an American way of life, *Antioch Rev.*, **13**, 131–54. Reprinted in: Wolfgang, M. E., et al., op. cit. (1962), pp. 213–25.

BENTHAM, J. (1838) *Principles of Penal Law*, II, 4, 4. In: *Works*, Edinburgh, **1**, 497–80.

BERGER, M. (1940) Murder, Inc. *Life* (1940), 30 Sept., pp. 86–88, 92–96. Reprinted in: Wolfgang, M. E., et al., op. cit. (1962), pp. 373–9.

BEYNON, E. D. (1934) Crimes and customs of the Hungarians in Detroit, *J. crim. Law Criminol.*, **25**, 755–74.

BIERSTEDT, R. (1964) art. Anomy (Anomie). In: Gould, J., and Kolb, W. L. (eds.), *A Dictionary of the Social Sciences*, London and New York, pp. 29–30.

BLANCHARD, W. H. (1959) The group process in gang rape, *J. soc. Psychol.*, **49**, 259–66.

BLOCH, H. A., and NIEDERHOFFER, A. (1958) *The Gang: A Study on Adolescent Behaviour*, New York.

BOHANNAN, P. (ed.) (1960) *African Homicide and Suicide*, Princeton, New Jersey.

BOND, I. K., and HUTCHISON, H. C. (1960) Application of reciprocal inihibition therapy to exhibitionism, *Canad. med. Assoc. J.*, **83**, 23–25.

BONDY, C., et al. (1957) *Jugendliche stören die Ordnung: Bericht und Stellungnahme zu den Halbstarkenkrawallen* [Young People disturb the Peace: Report and Appraisal of the Teenage Riots], Munich.

BORDUA, D. J. (1961) Delinquent subcultures: Sociological interpretations of gang delinquency, *Ann. Amer. Acad. polit. soc. Sci.*, **338**, 120–36. Reprinted in: Wolfgang, M. E., et al., op. cit. (1962), pp. 289–301 (A Critique of Sociological Interpretations of Gang Delinquency).

REFERENCES

BORINSKI, F., and MILCH, W. (1945) *Jugendbewegung: The Story of German Youth, 1896–1933* (German Educational Reconstruction, No. 3/4), London.

BOSLOW, H. M., ROSENTHAL, D., and GLIEDMAN, L. H. (1959) The Maryland Defective Delinquency Law, *Brit. J. Delinq.*, **10**, 5–13.

BOURCHIER, J. D. (1910) art. Albania, *Encycl. Brit.*, 11th ed., **1**, 484.

BOVET, L. (1951) *Psychiatric Aspects of Juvenile Delinquency*, World Health Org. Monogr. Ser., No. 1, Geneva. Cf. especially: pp. 8–10, 79 (Concept of Juvenile Delinquency), 55 (Chinese in U.S.).

BREARLY, H. C. (1932) *Homicide in the United States*, Chapel Hill, N. Carolina.

BRITISH MEDICAL ASSOCIATION (1964) *Venereal Disease and Young People: A Report by a Committee of the British Medical Association*, London, pp. 23–25 (Effect of Immigration).

British Medical Journal (1964) [Leading articles] Pep pill menace; Control of pep pills, *Brit. med. J.*, **1**, 792, 925.

BRONGERSMA, L. (1964) Revision of criminal law in Morocco, *Excerpta criminol.*, **4**, 267–72.

BUENO ARUS, F. (1962) La criminalidad en España, *Rev. Estud. penitenc.*, **18**, 48–51. English abstract in: *Excerpta criminol.*, 1963, **3**, 375.

BUJAN, B. (1961) Decrease of vendetta in the Macedonian People's Republic (Paper presented at 5th Congress Int. Acad. Legal Med. and Social Med., Vienna, May 1961). English abstract in: *Excerpta criminol.*, **1**, 193.

CALLAGAN, J. E. (1961) Survey of juvenile delinquency in Ontario (Paper presented at 3rd Biennial Canadian Congress of Corrections, Toronto, May 1961). Abstract in: *Excerpta criminol.*, **1**, 523.

CARAVEDO, B. (1959) Social Psychiatry in Peru. In: Masserman, J. H., and Moreno, J. L. (eds.), *Progress in Psychotherapy*, New York, **4**, 321.

CAUDILL, W. (1958) *The Psychiatric Hospital as a Small Society*, Cambridge, Mass.

CHAFETZ, M. E., and DEMONE, JR., H. W. (1962) *Alcoholism and Society*, New York.

CHEIN, I., et al. (1964) *Narcotics, Delinquency, and Social Policy: The Road to H*, London and New York.

CHEVERS, N. (1870) *A Manual of Medical Jurisprudence for India*, Calcutta, pp. 7–9, 148–50, 576–78.

CHRISTIANSEN, K. O. (1955) *Landssvigerkriminaliteten i sociologisk belysning* [The Criminality of Traitors in Sociological Perspective], Copenhagen. Cf. especially: Chap. 5.

CHRISTIANSEN, K. O. (1959) *Ungdomskriminaliteten i Danmark, 1933–55* [Juvenile Delinquency in Denmark, 1933–55] (Report Crim. Law Commission on Juvenile Delinquency), Copenhagen. English abstract in: *Excerpta criminol.*, 1961, **1**, 25.

—— (1960) Industrialization and urbanization in relation to crime and juvenile delinquency, *Int. Rev. crim. Policy*, **16**, 3–8.

—— (1964) Delinquent generations in Denmark: A Danish evaluation of Leslie T. Wilkins' methods and findings, *Brit. J. Criminol.*, **4**, 259–64.

CHURCH [OF ENGLAND] INFORMATION BOARD (1956) *Sexual Offenders and Social Punishment* (ed. D. S. Bailey), London.

CHURCH [OF ENGLAND] INFORMATION OFFICE (1959) *Ought Suicide to be a Crime? A Discussion of Suicide, Attempted Suicide and the Law*, London.

CHUTE, M. (1964) The London that was Shakespeare's, *UNESCO Courier*, **17** (May), 14–23. From: *Shakespeare of London*, by M. Chute, London and New York.

CLIFFORD, W. (1954) Delinquency in Cyprus, *Brit. J. Delinq.*, **5**, 146–50.

—— (1964) The African view of crime, *Brit. J. Criminol.*, **4**, 477–86.

CLINARD, M. B. (1962) Contributions of sociology to understanding deviant behaviour, *Brit. J. Criminol.*, **3**, 110–29.

CLOWARD, R. A. (1959) Illegitimate means, anomie, and deviant behaviour, *Amer. sociol. Rev.*, **24**, 164–76.

CLOWARD, R. A., and OHLIN, L. E. (1961) *Delinquency and Opportunity: A Theory of Delinquent Gangs*, Glencoe, Illinois.

COHEN, A. K. (1955) *Delinquent Boys: The Culture of the Gang*, Glencoe, Illinois. Cf. especially: pp. 24–32 (The Content of the Delinquent Subculture). (Also published: London, 1956).

COHEN OF BIRKENHEAD, Lord (1958) Epilepsy as a social problem, *Brit. med. J.*, **1**, 672–5.

COLIN, M., and BOURJADE, G. (1961) Les attentats aux moeurs dans les bandes d'adolescents – Essai de description criminologique d'une nouvelle figure sociopathique représentée par les attentats aux moeurs et viols collectifs réalisés au sein des bandes d'adolescents et de blousons noirs, *Ann. Méd. lég.*, **41**, 59–62.

CONNELL, P. H. (1958) *Amphetamine Psychosis* (Maudsley Monogr. No. 5), London.

—— (1964) Amphetamine misuse, *Brit. J. Addiction*, **60**, 9–27.

CRESSEY, D. R. (1960) Epidemiology and individual conduct: A case from criminology, *Pacific sociol. Rev.*, **3**, 47–54. Reprinted in: Wolfgang, M. E., et al., op. cit. (1962), pp. 81–90 (The Development of a Theory: Differential Association).

REFERENCES

CRESSEY, D. R. (1964) *Delinquency, Crime and Differential Association*, The Hague.

DAVIDSON, J. (1911) art. Dacoity, *Encycl. Religion and Ethics*, **4**, 384–5.

DAVIS, A., and DOLLARD, J. (1940) *Children of Bondage*, Washington, D.C.

DE QUINCEY, T. (1856) *Confessions of an English Opium-Eater*, Pt. II. In: *Works*, Edinburgh and London, **5**.

DE VOS, G. A., and MIZUSHIMA, K. (1959) *Organization and Social Function of Japanese Gangs: Some Parallels to the American Scene*, Univ. of Calif., Berkeley, Calif. (Unpublished, duplicated document.)

—— (1960) *Research on Delinquency in Japan: An Introductory Review*, Univ. of Calif., Berkeley, Calif. (Unpublished, duplicated document.)

—— (1962) The school and delinquency: Perspectives from Japan, *Teachers College Record*, **63**, 626–38.

DICKS, H. V. (1944–5) Reports to the Directorate of Army Psychiatry, War Office, London: *The Psychological Foundations of the Wehrmacht; Desertion in the German Forces;* and *National Socialism as a Psychologial Problem.* (Unpublished, duplicated departmental documents.)

—— (1947) In: Rees, J. R. (ed.), *The Case of Rudolf Hess*, London, pp. 195–202.

DUBOIS, J. A. (1905) *Hindu Manners, Customs and Ceremonies* (transl. and ed. H. K. Beauchamp – from French MS. of 1818), 3rd ed., Oxford, pp. 66–70.

†DULPHY, G., and GAUD, M. (eds.) (1959) *Etudes des Conditions de Vie de l'Enfant africain en Milieu urbain et de leur Influence sur la Délinquance juvénile* (Centre Int. de l'Enfance, Travaux et Documents, XII), Paris.

DURKHEIM, E. (1895) *Les Règles de la Méthode sociologique*, Paris. English transl. (8th ed.), *The Rules of Sociological Method* (ed. G. E. G. Catlin), Glencoe, Illinois, 1950. Cf. especially: pp. 65–73 (The Normal and the Pathological).

—— (1897) *Le Suicide: Etude de Sociologie*, Paris. English transl., *Suicide: A Study in Sociology* (ed. G. Simpson), Glencoe, Illinois, 1951; London, 1952.

EATON, J. W., and WEIL, R. J. (1955) *Culture and Mental Disorders: A Comparative Study of the Hutterites and Other Populations*, Glencoe, Illinois. Cf. especially: pp. 137–48, 188–207.

†ECOSOC (U.N.) (1964) *La Délinquance juvénile et la Rapidité des Changements sociaux en Afrique* (Paper prepared for Regional Meeting on Social Defence, Monrovia, August 1964 – Duplicated document: E/CN. 14/SODE/4).

*EISENSTADT, S. N. (1951) Delinquent group-formation among immigrant youth, *Brit. J. Delinq.*, **2**, 34–45.

—— (1954) *The Absorption of Immigrants*, London.

ELIADE, M. (1951) *Le Chamanisme et les Techniques archaïques de l'Extase*, Paris.

ELLIS, H. (1936) *Studies in the Psychology of Sex*, New York, **2**, Pt. 2, *Sexual Inversion*, Chap. 4, pp. 195–263.

EMPEY, L. T., and RABOW, J. (1961) The Provo Experiment in delinquency rehabilitation, *Amer. sociol. Rev.*, **26**, 679–95.

EYNON, T. G., and RECKLESS, W. C. (1961) Companionship at delinquency onset, *Brit. J. Criminol.*, **2**, 162–70.

EYSENCK, H. J. (1964) *Crime and Personality*, London.

FANDIÑO, P. J. J. (1962) Delincuencia juvenil, *Criminalia*, **28**, 296–308. English abstract in: *Excerpta criminol.*, 1963, **3**, 171.

FARQUHAR, J. N. (1921) art. Thags, *Encycl. Religion and Ethics*, **12**, 259–61.

FAUCONNET, P. (1928) *La Responsabilité: Etude de Sociologie*, 2nd ed., Paris.

FÉLICE, P. de (1936) *Poisons sacrés, Ivresses divines: Essai sur quelques Formes inférieures de la Mystique*, Paris.

FERRACUTI, F., and WOLFGANG, M. E. (1963) Design for a proposed study of violence: A socio-psychological study of a subculture of violence, *Arch. Criminol. Neuropsiq.*, **11**, 23–43. Reprinted in: *Brit. J. Criminol.*, 1963, **3**, 377–88.

—— (1964) Clinical v. sociological criminology: Separation or integration? *Excerpta criminol.*, **4**, 407–10.

FIELD, M. J. (1937) *Religion and Medicine of the Gã People*, Oxford.

—— (1955) Alcoholism, crime and delinquency in Soviet society, *Social Problems*, **3**, 100–9.

Field, The, London (1964), **223**, (May 14), 932.

FORAN, E. T. (1962) Narcotic addiction and the teenager, *Amer. J. Correction*, **24**, 8–12.

FRANCHINI, A., and INTRONA, F. (1961) *Delinquenza minorile: Problemi medico-legali, psicologici e giuridico-sociali* [Juvenile Delinquency: Medico-legal, Psychological and Socio-legal Probems], Padova. Cf. especially: pp. 125–35 (Socio-cultural environment), 457–87 (Statistics – including Internal Migration), 547–67 (Juvenile Gangs).

REFERENCES

FREDRIKSSON, G. (1962) *Kriminalstatistiken och Kriminologien* [Criminal Statistics and Criminology], Stockholm [in Swedish].

FREUND, K. (1960) Some Problems in the Treatment of Homosexuality, In: Eysenck, H. J. (ed.), *Behaviour Therapy and the Neuroses*, Oxford, pp. 312–26.

GAMIO, M. (1935) *Hacia un Mexico Nuevo: Problemas sociales* [Towards a New Mexico: Social Problems], Mexico City, pp. 186–7.

GELDER, M. G. (1965) Can behaviour therapy contribute to the treatment of delinquency? *Brit. J. Criminol.*, **5**, 365–76.

—— et al. (1964) Behaviour therapy and psychotherapy for phobic disorders (Paper presented at 6th Int. Congress of Psychotherapy, London).

GIBBENS, T. C. N. (1961) *Trends in Juvenile Delinquency*, World Health Org. Public Health Papers, No. 5, Geneva.

—— (1963) *Psychiatric Studies of Borstal Lads* (Maudsley Monogr. No. 11), London.

GIBBENS, T. C. N., and PRINCE, J. (1962) *Shoplifting*, London.

GIBBENS, T. C. N., and SILBERMAN, M. (1960) The clients of prostitutes, *Brit. J. vener. Dis.*, **36**, 113–17.

—— (in press) *Short-term offenders*, London.

GIBBENS, T. C. N., and WALKER, A. (1956) Violent cruelty to children, *Brit. J. Deling.*, **6**, 260–77.

GLUECK, S., and GLUECK, E. T. (1940) *Juvenile Delinquents Grown Up*, New York.

—— (1945) *After-Conduct of Discharged Offenders*, New York and London.

—— (1950) *Unravelling Juvenile Delinquency*, New York.

GORDON, M. M. (1947) The concept of the subculture and its application, *Social Forces*, **26**, 40–42

GRANT, J. D., and GRANT, M. Q. (1959) Group dynamics approach to the treatment of non-conformists in the Navy, *Ann. Amer. Acad. polit. soc. Sci.*, **322**, 126–35.

GRAY, L. H., et al. (1909) art. Blood-Feud, *Encycl. Religion and Ethics*, **2**, 720–35.

GREENBLATT, M., et al. (1955) *From Custodial to Therapeutic Patient Care in Mental Hospitals*, New York.

GRINDER, R. E., and MCMICHAEL, R. E. (1963) Cultural influence on conscience development: Resistance to temptation and guilt among Samoans and American Caucasians, *J. abnorm. soc. Psychol.*, **66**, 503–7.

GRYGIER, T., JONES, H., and SPENCER, C. (eds.) (1965) *Criminology in Transition*, London.

183

GUZMAN, S. (1962) Delincuencia y problemas médico-psicológicos del adolescente, *Rev. colomb. Pediat.*, **20**, 50–53. English abstract in: *Excerpta criminol.*, 1963, **3**, 172.

HALL WILLIAMS, J. E. (1964) art. Crime. In: Gould, J., and Kolb, W. L. (eds.) *A Dictionary of the Social Sciences*, London and New York, pp. 147–8.

HARMS, E. (1962) Drug addiction wave among adolescents, *New York State J. Med.*, **62**, 3996–7.

HARTWICH, C. (1911) *Die menschlichen Genussmittel* [The Euphoriant Drugs of Mankind], Leipzig.

HAYNER, N. S. (1942) Five Cities of the Pacific Northwest, In: Shaw, C. R., and McKay, H. D., op. cit. (1942), Chap. 16, pp. 353–87.

HAYNER, N. S., and REYNOLDS, C. N. (1933) Delinquency areas in the Puget Sound region, *Amer. J. Sociol.*, **39**, 314–28

HECKETHORN, C. W. (1897) *Secret Societies of All Ages and Countries*, 2nd ed., London, **1**, 264–81.

HEUYER, G. (1954) L'homosexualité: Conséquence de vagabondage, *Rev. Neuropsychiat. infantile*, **2**, 278–83.

HIRSCHFELD, M. (1914). *Die Homosexualität des Mannes und des Weibes* [Male and Female Homosexuality], Berlin, pp. 841–72 (Vergleichende Uebersicht der antihomosexuellen Strafgesetze) [Comparative Survey of the Penal Laws against Homosexuality].

HOLLINGSHEAD, A. B., and REDLICH, F. C. (1958) *Social Class and Mental Illness*, New York.

HOME OFFICE (ENGLAND) (1934) *Criminal Statistics: England and Wales, 1934*, London, pp. ix, xiii–xv.

—— (1957) *Report of the Committee on Homosexual Offences and Prostitution*, London.

HOOD, R. (1962) *Sentencing in Magistrates' Courts*, London.

HOWARD, J. (1784) *The State of the Prisons in England and Wales*, 3rd ed., Warrington, pp. 10–11.

HSU, F. L. K., et al. (1961) Culture patterns and adolescent behaviour, *Int. J. soc. Psychiat.*, **7**, 33–53.

HUNDERTMARK, D. (1962) Jugendkriminalität und Minderjährigenschutzgerichte in Spanien [Juvenile delinquency and courts for the protection of minors in Spain], *Recht der Jugend*, **10**, 113–18. English abstract in: *Excerpta criminol.*, **2**, 728.

HURSTON, Z. (1939) *Voodoo Gods: An Inquiry into Native Myths and Magic in Jamaica and Haiti*, London, pp. 203–9.

HUTCHISON, R. (1934) The barbiturates, *Lancet*, **1**, 481.

IGA, M. (1961) Cultural factors in suicides of Japanese youth with focus on personality, *Sociol. social Res.*, **46**, 75–90.

INTERPOL (1960) *Special Police Departments for the Prevention of Juvenile Delinquency*, Paris.
—— (1963) *International Crime Statistics, 1959–1960*, Paris.
—— (1964) *International Crime Statistics, 1961–1962*, Paris.
JANET, P. (1925) *Psychological Healing: A Historical and Clinical Study* (transl. from French), London and New York, 2 vols.
JASINSKI, J. (1962) *Juvenile and Young Adult Delinquents in Poland between the Years 1951 and 1962*, Dept. of Criminol., Inst. of Legal Sciences, Polish Acad. Sci., Warsaw. (Unpublished paper.)
JELLINEK, E. M. (1960) *The Disease Concept of Alcoholism*, New Haven, Conn., Chaps. 2 and 3.
JENKINS, R. L. (1949) The Psychopathic Delinquent. In: *Social Work in the Current Scene: Selected Papers* (76th Annual Meeting, National Conference of Social Work, June 1949), New York, 1950.
JOHNSON, A. (1959) Juvenile Delinquency, In: Arieti, S. (ed.), *American Handbook of Psychiatry*, New York, **1**, 840–56.
JOHNSON, G. B. (1941) The Negro and crime, *Ann. Amer. Acad. polit. soc. Sci.*, **271**, 93–104. Reprinted in: Wolfgang, M. E., et al., op. cit. (1962), pp. 145–53.
JONES, E. (1923) The Island of Ireland. In: *Essays in Applied Psycho-Analysis*, London, Chap. 12, pp. 398–414.
JONES, M., et al. (1952) *Social Psychiatry: A Study of Therapeutic Communities*, London.
—— et al. (1959) The psychopath and the Mental Health Bill, *Lancet*, **1**, 566–8.
JONES, V. C. (1948) *The Hatfields and the McCoys*, Chapel Hill, N. Carolina.
†JUNOD, H.-P. (1962) L'importance de quelques conceptions pénales africaines au moment de l'indépendance des états africains, *Acta Africana*, Geneva, **1**, 176–8. English abstract in: *Excerpta criminol.*, 1964, **4**, 120.
KARLSSON, B. (1963) Thinner-, alkohol- och tablettmissbruk bland barn och ungdom: Toxikologiska synpunkter [Thinner, alcohol and drug addiction in children and adolescents: Toxicological aspects], *Nord. Med.*, **70**, 893–6 (with English abstract).
KINSEY, A. C., et al. (1948) *Sexual Behaviour in the Human Male*, Philadelphia, pp. 274, 384–93.
KISKER, G. W. (ed.) (1951) *World Tension: The Psychopathology of International Relations*, New York.
KLINEBERG, O. (1940) *Social Psychology*, New York.
—— (1950) *Tensions Affecting International Understanding: A Survey of Research*, New York Soc. Sci. Res. Council, New York.

KLUCKHOHN, C. (1964) art. Culture. In: Gould, J., and Kolb, W. L. (eds.), *A Dictionary of the Social Sciences*, London and New York, pp. 165–8.

KOBRIN, S. (1951) The conflict of values in delinquency areas, *Amer. sociol. Rev.*, **16**, 653–61. Reprinted in: Wolfgang, M. E., et al., op. cit. (1962), pp. 259–66.

KOENIG, S. (1961) The Immigrant and Crime. In: Roucek, J. S. (ed.), *Sociology of Crime*, New York, pp. 138–59.

KVARACEUS, W. C. (1964) *Juvenile Delinquency: A Problem for the Modern World*, UNESCO, Paris.

LACASSAGNE, A. (1886) [Contributions to Congrès d'Anthropologie Criminelle, Rome, Nov. 1886—summary report]. *Arch. Anthropol. crim.*, **1**, 181–5.

LANDER, B. (1954) *Towards an Understanding of Juvenile Delinquency*, New York. Cf. especially: pp. 77–90 (An Ecological Analysis of Baltimore), reprinted in: Wolfgang, M. E., et al., op. cit. (1962), pp. 184–90.

LANDERS, J., MACPHAIL, D. S., and SIMPSON, R. C. (1954) Group therapy in H.M. Prison, Wormwood Scrubs: The application of analytical psychology, *J. ment. Sci.*, **100**, 953–60.

LANDIS, J. R., DINITZ, S., and RECKLESS, W. C. (1963) Implementing two theories of delinquency: Value orientation and awareness of limited opportunity, *Sociol. social Res.*, **47**, 408–16.

LAURENT, J.-M. (1962) Toxique et toxicomanie peu connus: 'Le cath', *Ann. méd.-psychol.*, **120**, 649–57.

LAVALLÉE, C., and MAILLOUX, N. (1964) Mécanismes de défense caractéristiques des groupes de jeunes délinquants en cours de rééducation, *Canad. J. Corrections*, **6**, 30–43.

LEE, R. H. (1952) Delinquent, neglected and dependent Chinese boys and girls of the San Francisco Bay region, *J. soc. Psychol.*, **36**, 15–34.

LEWIN, L. (1931) *Phantastica: Narcotic and Stimulating Drugs – Their Use and Abuse* (transl. from 2nd German ed.), London.

LEWIS, N. (1964) *The Honoured Society: The Mafia Conspiracy Observed*, London (pp. 22, 24–25, 32–33 cited).

Life (1963) art. 'The white devil's day is almost over', *Life*, **35**, No. 5 (9 Sept.), 23–30.

LIN, T. (1958) Tai-pau and Liu-mang: Two types of delinquent youth in Chinese society. In: *Growing Up in a Changing World*, World Fed. Mental Health, London, pp. 148–63. Reprinted in: *Brit. J. Deling.*, 1958, 8, 244–56; and in: Opler, M. K. (ed.), *Culture and Mental Health*, New York, 1959, pp. 257–71.

LIN, T., and STANDLEY, C. C. (1962) *The Scope of Epidemiology in Psychiatry*, World Health Org. Public Health Papers, No. 16, Geneva.

LINCOLN, C. E. (1964) *My Face is Black*, New York.

LIND, A. W. (1930) Some ecological patterns of community disorganization in Honolulu, *Amer. J. Sociol.*, **36**, 206–20.

LOGAN, R. F. L., and GOLDBERG, E. M. (1953) Rising eighteen in a London suburb: A study of some aspects of the life and health of young men, *Brit. J. Sociol.*, **4**, 323–45.

LOWES DICKINSON, G. (1945) *The Greek View of Life*, London, pp. 103–12.

MACIVER, R. M. (1950) *The Ramparts We Guard*, New York, p. 77.

MACKWOOD, J. C. (1949) The psychological treatment of offenders in prison, *Brit. J. Psychol.*, **40**, 5–22.

MAIER, N. R. F. (1949) *Frustration: The Study of Behaviour without a Goal*, New York.

MAILLOUX, N., and LAVALLÉE, C. (1960) Les attitudes sociales du jeune délinquant et le travail de la rééducation, *Rev. canad. Criminol.*, **2**, 185–96.

—— (1962) Genèse et signification de la conduite 'antisociale', *Rev. canad. Criminol.*, **4**, 103–11. English transl.: The genesis and meaning of 'anti-social' conduct, *Contributions à l'Etude des Sciences de l'Homme*, 1962, **5**, 158–67.

MANCINI, J.-G. (1962) *Prostitution et Proxénétisme*, Paris. English transl.: *Prostitutes and their Parasites*, London, 1963.

MANNHEIM, H. (1940) *Social Aspects of Crime in England between the Wars*, London.

—— (1942) Trends in the Incidence of Juvenile Delinquency. In: Carr-Saunders, A. M., et al., *Young Offenders: An Enquiry into Juvenile Delinquency*, Cambridge, Chap. 2, pp. 43–53.

MANSHARDT, C. (1959) *The Delinquent Child in India*, Bombay.

MARGOLIOUTH, D. S. (1909) art. Assassins. *Encycl. Religion and Ethics*, **2**, 138–41.

MARQUART, D. I. (1948) The pattern of punishment and its relation to abnormal fixation in adult human subjects, *J. general Psychol.*, **39**, 107–44.

MARTIN, J. M. (1961) *Juvenile Vandalism: A Study of its Nature and Prevention*, Springfield, Illinois.

MAYS, J. B. (1954) *Growing Up in the City: A Study of Juvenile Delinquency in an Urban Neighbourhood*, Liverpool.

MCCLINTOCK, F. H., and GIBSON, E. (1961) *Robbery in London*, London and New York.

McClintock, F. H., et al. (1963) *Crimes of Violence*, London and New York.

McCord, W., and McCord, J. (1959) *Origins of Crime: A New Evaluation of the Cambridge-Somerville Youth Study*, New York.

McCorkle, L. W. (1952) Group therapy in the treatment of offenders, *Fed. Probation*, **16**, 22–27.

McCorkle, L. W., and Korn, R. R. (1954) Resocialization within walls, *Ann. Amer. Acad. polit. soc. Sci.*, **293**, 88–98.

McGee, R. A. (1962) Youth and dangerous drugs, *Calif. Youth Authority Quart.*, **15**, 2.

Mead, M. (1935) *Sex and Temperament in Three Primitive Societies*, New York and London.

——— (1956) *New Lives for Old: Cultural Transformation – Manus, 1928–1953*, New York and London.

Meade, J. E., et al. (1961) *The Economic and Social Structure of Mauritius*, London.

Mecír, J. (1961) The influence of adolescent groups on the consumption of alcoholic drinks by minors. [Original art. in Czech, in *Cesk. Psychiat.*, **57**, 16–21.] *Excerpta criminol.*, **1**, 225 (English abstract).

Meige, H., and Feindel, E. (1907) *Tics and their Treatment* (transl. from French and ed. S. A. K. Wilson), London.

Merton, R. K. (1938) Social structure and anomie, *Amer. sociol. Rev.*, **3**, 672–82. Reprinted in: Wolfgang, M. E., et al., op. cit. (1962), pp. 236–43.

Merton, R. K., and Nisbet, R. A. (eds.) (1963) *Contemporary Social Problems: An Introduction to the Sociology of Deviant Behaviour and Social Disorganization*, New York.

Métraux, R., and Abel, T. M. (1957) Normal and deviant behaviour in a peasant community: Montserrat, B. W. I., *Amer. J. Orthopsychiat.*, **27**, 167–84.

Meyer, V., and Gelder, M. G. (1963) Behaviour therapy and phobic disorders, *Brit. J. Psychiat.*, **109**, 19–28.

Michaux, L., Duché, D. J., and Nodot, A. (1957) Histoire d'un gang d'enfants: Rôle de l'érotisme homosexuel dans la formation et le symbolisme des groupes d'enfants. *Rev. Neuropsychiat. infantile*, **5**, 392–6.

Middendorff, W. (1960) *New Forms of Juvenile Delinquency: Their Origin, Prevention and Treatment – General Report* (2nd U.N. Congress on Prevention of Crime and Treatment of Offenders, London, 1960), New York.

REFERENCES

MILLER, W. B. (1958) Lower class culture as a generating milieu of gang delinquency, *J. soc. Issues*, **14**, 5–19. Reprinted in: Wolfgang, M. W., et al., op. cit. (1962), pp. 267–76.

—— (1959) Preventive work with street-corner groups: Boston Delinquency Project, *Ann. Amer. Acad. polit. soc. Sci.*, **322**, 97–106.

*MILLO, E. (1960a) Juvenile Delinquency in Israel. In : Smilansky, M. (ed.), *Child and Youth Welfare in Israel*, Henrietta Szold Inst., Jerusalem, Israel, pp. 245–59.

*—— (1960b) *Prevention of Types of Criminality Resulting from Social Changes and Accompanying Economic Development in Less Developed Countries*, Ministry of Social Welfare, Jerusalem, Israel.

MINISTRY OF EDUCATION (INDIA) (1954) *Report on Delinquent Children and Juvenile Offenders in India*, New Delhi.

MINISTRY OF JUSTICE (JAPAN) (1963) *Summary of the White Paper on Crime, 1963*, Tokyo [in English].

MORENO, J. (1946) *Psychodrama*, New York.

MORRIS, T., and MORRIS, P. (1963) *Pentonville: A Sociological Study of an English Prison*, London.

MOSES, E. R. (1947) Differentials in crime rates between Negroes and Whites based on comparisons of four socio-economically equated areas, *Amer. sociol. Rev.*, **12**, 411–20. Reprinted in: Wolfgang, M. E., et al., op. cit., (1962), pp. 154–62.

MURPHY, H. B. M. (1963) Juvenile delinquency in Singapore, *J. soc. Psychol.*, **61**, 201–31.

NAIDU, M. P. (1912) *The History of Professional Poisoners and Coiners in India*, Madras, pp. 1–83.

NAKA, S. (1956) The Awaking-drug Addiction among Japanese Children and Young People, In: *Mental Health in Home and School*, World Fed. Mental Health, London, pp. 194–200.

NATIONAL COUNCIL ON CRIME AND DELINQUENCY (1963) Parliament orders Mafia probe, *Nat. Council Crime Delinq. News*, **9**, No. 2.

NORWEGIAN JOINT COMMITTEE ON INTERNATIONAL SOCIAL POLICY (1960) Treatment of offenders in Norway, *Canad. J. Corrections*, **2**, 358–62.

NYLANDER, I. (1963) Thinner-, alkohol- och tablettmissbruk bland barn och ungdom: Kliniska synpunkter [Thinner, alcohol and drug addiction in children and adolescents: Clinical aspects], *Nord. Med.*, **70**, 896–9 (with English abstract).

O'BRIEN, J. A. (ed.) (1954) *The Vanishing Irish: The Enigma of the Modern World*, London.

189

†ORTIGUES, M.-C., COLOT, A., and MONTAGNIER, M.-T. (1965) La délinquance juvénile à Dakar, *Psychopathol. africaine* (Bull. Soc. Psychopathol. Hyg. ment. Dakar), **1**, No. 1, 85–129.

OSWALD, I. (1962) Induction of illusory and hallucinatory voices with consideration of behaviour therapy, *J. ment. Sci.*, **108**, 196–212.

PARROT, P., and GUENEAU, M. (1960) Contribution à l'étude des gangs d'adolescents: Histoire d'une bande, *Ann. méd.-psychol.*, **2**, 837–62.

PARSONS, T. (1947) Certain primary sources and patterns of aggression in the social structure of the Western world, *Psychiatry* **10**, 167–81.

PATRICK, J. B. (1934) Studies in rational behaviour and emotional excitement—Pt. I: Rational behaviour in human subjects; Pt. II: The effect of emotional excitement on rational behaviour in human subjects, *J. compar. Psychol.*, **18**, 1–22; 153–95.

PATTERSON, S. (1963) *Dark Strangers: A Sociological Study of the Absorption of a Recent West Indian Migrant Group in Brixton, South London*, London and Bloomington, Indiana.

PAUL-PONT, I. (1956) Essai d'élaboration d'une méthode de recherche des facteurs de la délinquance juvénile dans les pays en voie de développement, *Courrier, Centre Int. de l'Enfance*, **6**, 311–20.

PAUL-PONT, I., and BELVÈZE, L. (1955) *Enquête sur la Délinquance juvénile en Afrique*, Centre Int. de l'Enfance, Paris. (Duplicated document.)

†PAUL-PONT, I., and FLIS, F. (1959) *Le Bien-être de l'Enfant en Afrique au Sud du Sahara* (Child Welfare in Africa South of the Sahara). (Colloque organisé par le C.I.E. et la C.C.T.A., Lagos, Nigeria, mars 1959). Centre Int. de l'Enfance, Paris.

PAYNE, R. B. (1963) Nutmeg intoxication, *New England J. Med.*, **269**, 36–38.

PEARCE, J. (1963) *Aspects of Transvestism.* (Unpublished M.D. Thesis, Univ. of London.)

PENROSE, L. S. (1949) *The Biology of Mental Defect*, London.

PERRY, E., and STONE, M. (1963) Impressions of the I.S.T.D. study tour to the U.S.S.R., *Brit. J. Criminol.*, **4**, 170–6.

†PIDOUX, C. (1956) Un conflit d'acculturation, *Acta psychother. psychosom. orthopaedag.*, **4**, 170–80.

PIERRE, E., FLAMAND, J.-P., and COLLOMB, H. (1963) La délinquance juvénile à Dakar, *Int. Rev. crim. Policy*, **20**, 27–33.

PITTMAN, D. J., and SNYDER, C. R. (eds.) (1962) *Society, Culture and Drinking Patterns*, New York and London.

POLLACK, O. (1950) *The Criminality of Women*, Philadelphia.

POND, D. A. (1961) Psychiatric aspects of epileptic and brain-damaged children, *Brit. med. J.*, **2**, 1377–82, 1454–9.

POWER, E. E. (1922) *Mediaeval English Nunneries*, Cambridge.

PRONK, B. (1961) Criminality in Surinam (Dutch Guiana), *Excerpta criminol.*, **1**, 485–94.

PRYS WILLIAMS, G. (1963) *Patterns of Teenage Delinquency.* Cited by: Walters, A. A., op. cit. (1963).

PULEO, G. (1962) La medicina sociale nella lotta contro un grave fenomeno sociale in Sicilia [Social medicine in the fight against a serious social manifestation in Sicily], *Difesa soc.*, **41**, 12–25. English abstract in: *Excerpta criminol.*, 1963, **3**, 277.

RACINE, A. (1959) *La Délinquance juvénile en Belgique de 1939 à 1957* (Centre d'Etude de la Délinquance Juvénile, Publ. No. 2), Brussels.

—— (1961) *La Délinquance juvénile en Belgique en 1958 et 1959* (Centre d'Etude de la Délinquance Juvénile, Publ. No. 7), Brussels.

RAMAN, A. C. (1960) The effect of rapid culture change on mental health, *World ment. Health*, **12**, 152–62.

—— (1962) The Eldest Child in Various Cultural Groups, *Report 1st Pan-African Psychiatric Conference*, Abeokuta, Nigeria, pp. 48–53.

RAMSBOTTOM, J. (1923) *A Handbook of the Larger British Fungi*, London, p. 26.

RATTRAY, R. S. (1923) *Ashanti*, London.

RAYMOND, M. J. (1956) Case of fetishism treated by aversion therapy, *Brit. med. J.*, **2**, 854–7.

RECKLESS, W. C. (1940) *Criminal Behavior*, New York, p. 112.

—— (1958) A self gradient among potential delinquents, *J. crim. Law Criminol.*, **49**, 230–3.

—— (1961a) A new theory of delinquency and crime, *Fed. Probation*, **25**, 42–46.

—— (1961b) Halttheorie [Containment theory], *Monatschr. Kriminol.*, **44**, 1–14.

—— (1961c) *The Crime Problem*, 3rd ed., New York, Chap. 18.

—— (1962) A non-causal explanation: Containment theory, *Excerpta criminol.*, **2**, 131–4.

RECKLESS, W. C., DINITZ, S., and MURRAY, E. (1956) Self concept as an insulator against delinquency, *Amer. sociol. Rev.*, **21**, 744–6.

—— (1957) The 'good' boy in a high delinquency area, *J. crim. Law Criminol.*, **48**, 18–26.

—— (1962) Self concept as a predictor of juvenile delinquency, *Amer. J. Orthopsychiat.*, **32**, 159–68.

RECKLESS, W. C., and SHOHAM, S. (1963) Norm containment theory as applied to delinquency and crime, *Excerpta criminol.*, **3**, 637–45.

REDL, F. (1945) The Psychology of Gang Formation and the Treatment of Juvenile Delinquents. In: *The Psychoanalytic Study of the Child*, New York and London, **1**, 367–77.

REID, D. D. (1960) *Epidemiological Methods in the Study of Mental Disorders*, World Health Org. Public Health Papers, No. 2. Geneva.

*REIFEN, D. (1955a) Juvenile delinquency and culture conflict in Israel, *Howard J.*, **9**, 130–6.

*—— (1955b) Juvenile delinquency in a changing society, *Jewish soc. Service Quart.*, **31**, 401–16.

—— (1960) *New Forms of Juvenile Delinquency in Israel: Their Origin, Prevention and Treatment*. (Paper prepared for 2nd U.N. Congress on Prevention of Crime and Treatment of Offenders – Unpublished, duplicated document.) Extracts in: Middendorff, W., op. cit. (1960), pp. 28–29, 30–31, 61–62.

*—— (1964a) *Patterns and Motivations of Juvenile Delinquency among Israeli Arabs*, Ministry of Social Welfare, Jerusalem, Israel.

*—— (1964b) Etude comparative de délinquants juvéniles juifs et arabes en Israël, *Rev. Droit pén. Criminol.*, **45**, 162–77.

REISS, A. J., JR., and RHODES, A. L. (1964) An empirical test of differential association theory, *J. Res. Crime Delinq.*, **1**, 5–18.

REPORT OF THE COMMITTEE FOR INVESTIGATING THE CAUSES OF THE ALARMING INCREASE OF JUVENILE DELINQUENCY IN THE METROPOLIS, London, 1816.

RETTIG, S., and PASAMANICK, B. (1960) Differences in the structure of moral values of students and alumni, *Amer. sociol. Rev.*, **25**, 550–5.

RICHELLE, M., et al. (1957) *Enfants Juifs Nord-Africains: Essai psycho-pédagogique à l'Intention des Éducateurs*, Tel-Aviv.

RIESMAN, D. (1950) *The Lonely Crowd: A Study of the Changing American Character*, New Haven, Conn., and London.

ROGOVIN, E. B. (1961) Social conformity and the comradely courts in the Soviet Union, *Crime and Delinq.*, **7**, 303–11.

ROSE, G. (1959) Status and grouping in a Borstal institution, *Brit. J. Delinq.*, **9**, 258–75.

ROSE, H. J. (1921) art. Suicide. *Encycl. Religion and Ethics*, **12**, 21–24.

ROSENWALD, R. J., and RUSSELL, D. H. (1961) Cough-syrup addiction, *New England J. Med.*, **264**, 927.

ROS JIMENO, J. (1961) Statistics in the service of the courts, *Rev. Obra Protec. Menores*, **18**, 27–42. Abstract in: *Excerpta criminol.*, 1962, **2**, 240.

ROUCEK, J. S. (1961) Crime in the U.S.S.R. and the European Satellites. In: Roucek, J. S. (ed.), *Sociology of Crime*, New York, pp. 427–545 – (incl. chapter on: Juvenile Delinquency and Crime in the Soviet Bloc, pp. 427–52).

ROUCH, J. (1963) Introduction à l'étude de la communauté de Bregbo, *J. Soc. Africanistes*, **33**, 129–202.

RUSSELL, M. (1964) The Irish Delinquent in England, Studies, Law Department, University of Dublin, June.

SAAVEDRA, E. B., and RAVE, G. M. (1963) Violencia política en Colombia, *Proc. 12th Int. Course Criminol.*, Jerusalem, Israel, **2**, Pt. 2, 358–70.

SAINSBURY, P. (1955) *Suicide in London: An Ecological Study* (Maudsley Monogr. No. 1), London.

SANFORD, N. (1963) *Report on Trip to Russia*, Univ. of Calif., Berkeley, Calif. (Unpublished, duplicated document.)

SARAN, A. R. (1962) Murder among the Munda: A case study, *Indian J. soc. Work,*, **23**, 1–7.

SARRÓ, R. (1961) The Promotion of Mental Health in Spain. In: Thornton, E. M. (ed.), *Planning and Action for Mental Health*, World Fed. Mental Health, London, pp. 27–28.

SAVITZ, L. (1962) Delinquency and Migration. (Originally issued as duplicated document, by Commission on Human Relations, Philadelphia, Jan. 1960.) In: Wolfgang, M. E., et al., op. cit. (1962), pp. 199–205.

SCARPITTI, F. R., et al. (1960) The 'good' boy in a high delinquency area: Four years later, *Amer. sociol. Rev.*, **25**, 555–8. Reprinted in: Wolfgang, M. E., et al., op. cit. (1962), pp. 206–9.

SCHRAG, C. (1954) Leadership among prison inmates, *Amer. sociol. Rev.*, **19**, 37–42.

SCOTT, P. D. (1956) Gangs and delinquent groups in London, *Brit. J. Delinq.*, **7**, 8–21. Reprinted in: Wolfgang, M. E., et al., op. cit. (1962), pp. 310–18.

—— (1960a) Assessing the offender for the courts: The role of the psychiatrist, *Brit. J. Criminol.*, **1**, 116–29.

—— (1960b) The treatment of psychopaths, *Brit. med. J.*, **1**, 1641–5.

—— (1964) Approved School success rates, *Brit. J. Criminol.*, **4**, 525–56.

SELLIN, T. (1938) *Culture Conflict and Crime* (Soc. Sci. Res. Council Bull. 41), New York. Also published in: *Amer. J. Sociol.*, 1938, **44**, 97–103.

—— (1940) *The Criminality of Youth*, Philadelphia.

SELLIN, T. (1951) The significance of records of crime, *Law Quart. Rev.*, **67**, 489–504. Reprinted in: Wolfgang, M. E., et al., op. cit. (1962), pp. 59–68.

—— (1963) Organized crime: A business enterprise, *Ann. New York Acad. Sci.*, **347**, 12–19.

SELLIN, T., and WOLFGANG, M. E. (1964) *The Measurement of Delinquency*, New York.

SETHNA, M. J. (1952) *Society and the Criminal, with special Reference to the Problems of Crime and its Prevention, the Personality of the Criminal, Prison Reform and Juvenile Delinquency in India*, Bombay – (Pt. 3 comprises a survey of juvenile delinquency in India).

*SHANAN, J. (1962) Cultural Waywardness as a Breeding-ground of Delinquency in Israel. (Paper presented at 12th Int. Course Criminol., Jerusalem, Israel, Sept. 1962). Abstract in: *Excerpta criminol.*, 1963, **3**, 158.

SHAW, C. R., and McKAY, H. D. (1942) *Juvenile Delinquency and Urban Areas: A Study of Rates of Delinquents in Relation to Differential Characteristics of Local Communities in American Cities*, Chicago. Cf. especially: Chap. 7, pp. 164–83 (Differences in Social Values and Organization among Local Communities), and pp. 435–41 (Summary and Interpretation).

SHOHAM, S. (1962) The application of the 'culture-conflict' hypothesis to the criminality of immigrants in Israel, *J. crim. Law. Criminol.*, **53**, 207–14.

*—— (1964) Conflict situations and delinquent solutions, *J. soc. Psychol.*, **64**, 185–215.

*SHOHAM, S., EREZ, R., and RECKLESS, W. C. (1964) Value orientation and awareness of differential opportunity of delinquent and non-delinquent boys in Israel, *Criminologica*, **2**, No. 3, 11–14.

SHOHAM, S., and HOVAV, M. (1964) B'nei-Tovim middle- and upper-class delinquency in Israel, *Sociol. social Res.*, **48**, 454–68.

SHORT, J. F., and STRODTBECK, F. L. (1964) Why gangs fight, *Transaction*, **1**, No. 6, 25–27.

SICOT, M. (1964) *La Prostitution dans le Monde*, Paris.

SIELICKA, M. (1961) Alcoholism among young people. [Original art. in Polish, in *Polski Tygodnik Lekarski*, **16**, 1907–9.] *Excerpta criminol.*, 1962, **2**, 423 (English abstract).

SIEMSEN, H. (1940) *Hitler Youth* (transl. from German), London, p. 118.

SLAVSON, S. K. (1951) Current trends in group psychotherapy, *Int. J. Group Psychother.*, **1**, 7–15.

REFERENCES

SLEEMAN, W. H. (1836) *Ramaseeana, or a Vocabulary of the Language used by the Thugs, with an Appendix descriptive of the Fraternity*, Calcutta. (Pp. 7–8 cited.)

SMITH, R. A. (1961) The incredible Electrical Conspiracy, *Fortune*, 1961, April, pp. 132–80; May, pp. 161–224. Reprinted in: Wolfgang, M. E., et al., op. cit. (1962), pp. 357–72.

SMITH, S. E. (1956) Fetishism treated by aversion therapy, *Brit. med. J.*, **2**, 1301–2.

SODDY, K. (ed.) (1955–6) *Mental Health and Infant Development*, London and New York, 2 vols.

—— (ed.) (1961) *Mental Health and Value Systems.* In: *Cross-cultural Studies in Mental Health*, London, pp. 57–172.

SPINLEY, B. M. (1953) *The Deprived and the Privileged*, London.

SRIVASTAVA, S. S. (1963) *Juvenile Vagrancy: A Socio-ecological Study of Juvenile Vagrants in the Cities of Kanpur and Lucknow*, London.

STENGEL, E. (1959) Classification of mental disorders, *Bull. World Health Org.*, **21**, 601–63.

STOFFLET, E. H. (1935) A Study of National and Cultural Differences in Criminal Tendency, *Arch. Psychol.*, No. 185, New York.

STÜRUP, G. (1952) The treatment of criminal psychopaths in Herstedvester, *Brit. J. med. Psychol.*, **25**, 31–38.

—— (1959) *Teamwork in the Treatment of Psychopathic Criminals*, Herstedvester.

SUTHERLAND, E. H. (1924) *Criminology*, 1st ed., Philadelphia.

—— (1940) White collar criminality, *Amer. sociol. Rev.*, **5**, 1–12.

—— (1941) Crime and business, *Ann. Amer. Acad. polit. soc. Sci.*, **217**, 112–18.

—— (1945) Is 'white collar crime' crime? *Amer. sociol. Rev.*, **10**, 132–9. Reprinted in: Wolfgang, M. E., et al., op. cit. (1962), pp. 20–27.

—— (1949) *White Collar Crime*, New York.

SUTHERLAND, E. H., and CRESSEY, D. R. (1955) *Principles of Criminology*, 5th ed., New York. Cf. especially: pp. 74–81.

SVERI, K. (1960) *Kriminalitet og Alder* [Crime and Age], Stockholm [in Norwegian].

SYKES, G. M. (1956) *Crime and Society*, New York.

—— (1958) *The Society of Captives*, Princeton, New Jersey.

SYKES, G. M., and MATZA, D. (1957) Techniques of neutralization: A theory of delinquency, *Amer. sociol. Rev.*, **22**, 664–70. Reprinted in: Wolfgang, M. E., et al., op. cit. (1962), pp. 249–54.

SYKES, G. M., and MESSINGER, S. L. (1960) *Theoretical Studies in the Social Organization of the Prison* (Soc. Sci. Res. Council Pamphlet No. 15), New York.

195

TAFT, D. R. (1942) *Criminology: An Attempt at a Synthetic Interpretation with Cultural Emphasis*, New York, Chap. 12, pp. 177–98 (Organized Crime).

TAIT, D. (1963) A sorcery hunt in Dagomba, *Africa*, London, **33**, 136–47.

TAKMAN, J. (1963) Thinner-, alkohol- och tablettmissbruk bland barn och ungdom: Socialmedicinska synpunkter [Thinner, alcohol and drug addiction in children and adolescents: Socio-medical aspects], *Nord. Med.*, **70**, 899–903 (with English abstract).

TANNER, J. M., and INHELDER, B. (eds.) (1956–60) *Discussions on Child Development*, London, 4 vols.

TAUXIER, L. (1932) *Religion, Mœurs et Coutumes des Agnis de la Côte d'Ivoire (Indénié et Sanwi)*, Paris.

THRASHER, F. M. (1927) *The Gang: A Study of 1,313 Gangs in Chicago*, Chicago.

TIEBOUT, H. M., and KIRKPATRICK, M. E. (1932) Psychiatric factors in stealing, *Amer. J. Orthopsychiat.*, **2**, 114–23.

TYLER, G. (1962a) *Organized Crime in America: A Book of Readings*, Ann Arbor, Mich.

—— (1962b) The roots of organized crime, *Crime and Delinq.*, **8**, 325–38.

—— (1963) An interdisciplinary attack on organized crime, *Ann. New York Acad. Sci.*, **347**, 104.

UNESCO (1956a) *The Race Question in Modern Science*, Paris. (Th whole work is important, but cf. especially: O. Klineberg, Race and Psychology, pp. 55–84, and A. M. Rose, The Roots of Prejudice, pp. 215–43.)

†—— (1956b) *Social Implications of Industrialization and Urbanization in Africa South of the Sahara*, Paris.

—— (1956c) *The Social Implications of Industrialization and Urbanization: Five Studies of Urban Populations of Recent Rural Origin in Cities of Southern Asia*, Calcutta.

—— (1957) *The Nature of Conflict: Studies on the Sociocultural Aspects of International Tensions*, Paris.

UNITED NATIONS (1956) *First United Nations Congress on the Prevention of Crime and the Treatment of Offenders* (Geneva, 1955) – *Report prepared by the Secretariat*, New York.

—— (1960) *New Forms of Juvenile Delinquency: Their Origin, Prevention and Treatment – Report prepared by the Secretariat* (2nd U.N. Congress on Prevention of Crime and Treatment of Offenders, London, 1960), New York. (Pp. 51–53 cited.)

URBAN, W. H. (1962) Suicide: A cultural and semantic view, *Ment. Hyg.*, New York, **46**, 377–81.

REFERENCES

VEILLARD-CYBULSKI, M. (1963) La délinquance juvénile en Suisse, *Schweiz. Zeitschr. Strafrecht*, **79**, 231–2.

VICTORIA, STATE OF (AUSTRALIA) (1956) *Report of Juvenile Delinquency Advisory Committee*, Melbourne, p. 54.

VIQUEIRA HINOJOSA, A. (1962) Criminalidad homosexual, *Criminalia*, **28**, 564–7. English abstract in: *Excerpta criminol.*, 1963, **3**, 575.

VOEGELE, G. E., and DIETZE, H. J. (1963) Addiction to gasoline smelling in juvenile delinquents, *Brit. J. Criminol.*, **4**, 43–60.

WALKER, N. (1965) *Crime and Punishment in Britain: The Penal System in Theory, Law and Practice*, Edinburgh.

WALTERS, A. A. (1963) Delinquent generations? *Brit. J. Criminol.*, **3**, 391–5.

WATT, L. (1961) Venereal disease in adolescents, *Brit. med. J.*, **2**, 858–60.

WEEKS, A. (1958) *Youthful Offenders at Highfields*, Ann Arbor, Mich.

WEST, D. J. (1963) *The Habitual Prisoner*, London and New York.

WESTERMARCK, E. (1906–8) *The Origin and Development of the Moral Ideas*, London, 2 vols.

—— (1932) *Ethical Relativity*, London.

—— (1939) *Christianity and Morals*, London.

WHARTON, K. (1964) The road to Clacton pier, *Spectator*, London, 1964 (3 Apr.), 444–5.

WHYTE, W. F. (1943) *Street Corner Society: The Social Structure of an Italian Slum*, Chicago.

WICKERSHAM, G. W., et al. (1933) *National Commission on Law Observance and Law Enforcement, Report No. 10*, Washington, D.C.

WILKINS, L. (1960) *Delinquent Generations* (Home Office: Studies in the Causes of Delinquency and the Treatment of Offenders, 3), London.

WILSON, H. C., and WILSON, A. J. C. (1964) Juvenile delinquency in Japan, *Brit. J. Criminol.*, **4**, 278–82.

WIRTH, L. (1931) Culture conflict and misconduct. *Social Forces*, **9**, 484–92.

WOETZEL, R. K. (1963) An overview of organized crime: Mores versus morality, *Ann. New York Acad. Sci.*, **347**, 1–11.

WOLFGANG, M. E., SAVITZ, L., and JOHNSTON, N. (eds.) (1962) *The Sociology of Crime and Delinquency*, New York.

WOLPE, J. (1958) *Psychotherapy by Reciprocal Inhibition*, Stanford, Calif.

WOOTTON, B. (1959) *Social Science and Social Pathology*, London.

WORLD FEDERATION FOR MENTAL HEALTH (1961) *Mental Health in International Perspective*, London. (Pp. 31–34, 47–48 cited.)

WORLD HEALTH ORGANIZATION (1961) *Programme Development in the Mental Health Field: 10th Report of the Expert Committee on Mental Health*, World Health Org. techn. Rep. Ser., 223, Geneva, pp. 33–34.

YABLONSKY, L. (1959) The delinquent gang as a near-group, *Social Problems*, **7**, 108–17. Reprinted in: Wolfgang, M. E., et al., op. cit. (1962), pp. 302–9.

—— (1962) *The Violent Gang*, New York.

YAP, P. M. (1958) *Suicide in Hong Kong*, Hong Kong.

INDEX